Imaging and Diagnosis in Pediatric Brain
Tumor Studies

Monika Warmuth-Metz

Imaging and Diagnosis in Pediatric Brain Tumor Studies

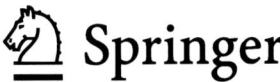 Springer

Monika Warmuth-Metz
Neuroradiology
Universityhospital Würzburg
Würzburg
Germany

Contributing author
Stefan Rutkowski
Department of Pediatric Oncology and Hematology
HIT-MED-Study Center
University Hospital of Hamburg Eppendorf
Hamburg
Germany

ISBN 978-3-319-42501-6   ISBN 978-3-319-42503-0   (eBook)
DOI 10.1007/978-3-319-42503-0

Library of Congress Control Number: 2016955081

Printed on acid-free paper

This Springer imprint is published by Springer Nature
The registered company is Springer International Publishing AG Switzerland
The registered company address is: Gewerbestrasse 11, 6330 Cham, Switzerland

Foreword

Once the modern era of neurosurgery began nearly a century ago, it became evident that a uniform system of classifying and grading brain tumors would be invaluable in guiding therapeutic decisions and comparing the relative efficacy of different treatment regimens. A number of schemas were adopted, some widely, some idiosyncratic, and others limited to one or a small group of institutions. No worldwide standard existed until the World Health Organization (WHO) began convening a panel of expert neuropathologists with the goal of developing a uniform, internationally-recognized system that could be applied across different institutions.

Beginning in 1986, the WHO Classification of CNS Neoplasms rapidly became the worldwide reference standard. It has been updated approximately every 7 years, with the fourth edition published in 2007 and the "4-plus" edition just published in May, 2016. Brain tumor trials that evaluate efficacy of different treatment regimens are largely based on the WHO classification system.

As imaging has become increasingly more sophisticated, it has become an integral part of brain tumor diagnosis and follow-up. The Reference Center for Imaging for the HIT-trials of the GPOH based at the University Hospital of Wurzburg is—to my knowledge—a unique resource for understanding imaging findings as they relate to brain tumor pathology. Where else would such a large repository of cases be found? Under the direction of the eminent pediatric neuroradiologist Dr. Monika Warmuth-Metz, the Reference Center assures uniform imaging evaluation and accurate diagnosis of brain tumors. This book is a unique, highly useful resource for radiologists who image brain tumors in children. With its emphasis on how to image neoplasms and then evaluate those images accurately and consistently, this guide is an essential addition to the neuroradiologist's bookshelf (whether print or electronic).

Anne G. Osborn, M.D.
University Distinguished Professor
William H. and Patricia W. Child Presidential Endowed Chair
University of Utah School of Medicine
Salt Lake City, Utah, USA

Acknowledgements

The German Reference Center for Imaging for the German brain tumor studies is supported by the German Childhood Cancer Foundation (Deutsche Kinderkrebsstiftung).

Contents

Chapter 1
The Impact of Staging Examinations in Children and Adolescents with Brain Tumor

Pediatric brain tumors, especially embryonal and other high-grade tumor types, have the propensity to disseminate along the cerebrospinal fluid (CSF) pathway, while spread outside the central nervous system (CNS) at diagnosis is very rare. The management of pediatric brain tumors has evolved over the last three decades as a result of prospective multicentric clinical trials. Multimodal treatment including surgical resection, radiotherapy, and chemotherapy has led to improved outcomes in many entities. However, treatment-related toxicity often has a major impact on long-term quality of survival. In order to reduce sequelae, the concept of stratification into risk groups according to clinical variables (e.g., age, presence of metastases detected by imaging or cytological evaluation of CSF, and postoperative residual tumor status) has been developed in the last decades, adjusting the intensity of therapy to the risk of relapse. While the principal treatment strategies have not significantly changed over the past few years, enormous progress has been made in understanding of tumor biology, which has led and most likely will continue to lead to further refinements of risk stratification and to the development of novel therapy approaches using targeted drugs in a personalized way [1].

1.1 Postoperative Residual Tumor

The aims of surgery are a maximum resection of the primary tumor with minimal damage of neurological function in order to reduce any mass effect, to debulk vital tumor tissue, to establish the biopathological diagnosis, and, if possible, to restore CSF flow. In view of the efficacy of the adjuvant treatment, a microsurgically complete resection should only be intended in case of tolerable risk, and dependent on the effectivity and risk of adjuvant treatment modalities.

To evaluate the extent of resection precisely with a low risk of artifacts, the postoperative MRI should be performed in the best technical way and timing possible. In case of significant residual tumor, particularly in nonmetastatic disease,

© Springer International Publishing Switzerland 2017
M. Warmuth-Metz, *Imaging and Diagnosis in Pediatric Brain Tumor Studies*,
DOI 10.1007/978-3-319-42503-0_1

second-look surgery should be discussed in some entities either directly after the primary operation or in the course of further treatment.

1.2   Metastases

For staging, the clinical classification according to the modified Chang system [2] has been generally accepted for medulloblastoma (MB), and is used accordingly in other brain tumors. It comprises an MRI examination of the full craniospinal axis and an evaluation of lumbar CSF cytology. As immediate postoperative assessment of CSF can yield false positive results due to surgical detritus, the optimum time-frame for lumbar puncture between surgery and start of adjuvant treatment should be used. In MB, it is commonly defined by day 14 after surgery. Artifacts and clinical needs should also be considered in the timing of postoperative cranial MRI and spinal MRI. Postoperative contrast enhancement (sometimes up to a few weeks) and post-functional MRI alterations (e.g., subdural enhancement) may be difficult to distinguish from metastases or laminar meningeal disease. Therefore, spinal MRI should be performed before lumbar puncture or – in case of suspicion of MB – ideally even before tumor surgery.

1.3   Risk-Adapted Treatment Stratification

Starting in the mid-twentieth century, the first decades of curative brain tumor treatment were characterized by a growing number of long-term survivors by means of gradual treatment intensification, albeit often at the price of a relevant impairment of quality of life. In the past two decades, with increasing knowledge on clinical risk factors, stratification of patients into different risk groups has allowed controlled de-escalation of treatment intensity within clinical trials.

It has been shown in various prospective trials for children with pediatric brain tumors that incomplete staging assessments are associated with adverse clinical outcome [3, 4]. Therefore, inadequate staging may lead either to undertreatment and lower survival rates, or overtreatment with potentially unnecessary treatment-induced late-effects, and must be avoided.

In addition, knowledge about biology of pediatric brain tumors has evolved faster than ever by the use of high-throughput methods for transcriptomics in the past few years. Most likely, biological classifications will continue to evolve, and further refined subgrouping has already been suggested.

The increasing knowledge of biologic heterogeneity of brain tumors [5] has led to a paradigm shift holding the promise of a much better tailored approach to risk stratification. Therefore, clinical risk factors (age, extent of resection, metastases) and biological factors (histology including histological subtypes, biological subgroups and signaling pathways, and prognostic genetic alterations, e.g., gene amplifications such as myc-amplification MB) will be used in increasingly refined algorithms for the different brain tumor entities in currently open and planned clinical trials.

In summary, clinical staging investigations must be considered as one of the very fundamental components of quality assessment in clinical care of children and adolescents with brain tumors. Results of present and future clinical trials will only be highly informative, if they are performed accurately and confirmed by central reference assessments.

Chapter 2
Structure of the Pediatric Competence Network of the German GPOH (Society of Pediatric Oncology and Hematology)

The pediatric oncologists in Germany are running multicenter treatment optimization studies for all kinds of tumors including CNS tumors. They have instituted reference centers for neuropathology, CSF cytology, radiotherapy, and neuroradiology for these studies in order to harmonize the individual results of histological diagnosis, staging, treatment, and response evaluation of their patients who are diagnosed and treated in many different hospitals all over the country [6, 7] rather than in few specialized centers. It has been recognized in several German and European studies that the event-free survival (EFS) of the study patients has been improved by a central review process [8]. The author has been working as the leader of the reference center for neuroradiology for more than 20 years. The aim of this publication is to present on one hand an easy way to approximately predict or sometimes diagnose the histology of many pediatric brain tumors from the aspect on imaging examinations, and on the other hand to guide into the different aspects of trial requirements, frequent diagnostic quality problems, and questions from the oncologists that have to be answered by the radiologist and are influencing the planning of imaging procedures.

Clearly, through the past years if not to say meanwhile decades magnetic resonance imaging (MRI) is dominating the imaging in all kinds of central nervous system (CNS) tumors. But certain features on computed tomography (CT) like the density of the solid parts of tumors, corresponding to the cell density on histological examination, bears indispensible information for the differential diagnosis. As the reference evaluation in the pediatric brain tumor trials is based on structural MRI, we will not cover multimodal imaging methods like diffusion tensor MRI, perfusion techniques, or MRI spectroscopy. We also will not cover positron emission tomography (PET) because this is a nuclear medicine method and beyond the scope of a neuroradiologist.

© Springer International Publishing Switzerland 2017
M. Warmuth-Metz, *Imaging and Diagnosis in Pediatric Brain Tumor Studies*,
DOI 10.1007/978-3-319-42503-0_2

Chapter 3
Imaging Differential Diagnosis of Pediatric CNS Tumors

3.1 Explanatory Note

After termination of this book the new WHO-classification of central nervous system tumors has been published [9]. As a completely new classification system frequently based on genetic definitions and no longer purely on histology has been created some entities in the following chapters have been abolished and do no longer exist like "gliomatosis cerebri". Others have been refined and are called now differently like "embryonal tumors with multilayered rosettes" (ETMR) for the former PNET.

"CNS embryonal tumor NOS" has to be used in the future for an AT/RT without the confirmation of the characteristic molecular defect.

As the present experience with the imaging characteristics of pediatric brain tumors is based on the last WHO-classification system published in 2007 only rarely experiences with some of the new entities like the genetically defined groups of MB exist. Further knowledge on imaging characteristics of the new entities will be acquired only in the future and has not yet been included in this book.

3.2 Embryonal Tumors

Embryonal tumors primarily affect children and only rarely adults. They are derived from embryonal cells and comprise the most frequent highly malignant tumors in children, like MBs, primitive neuroectodermal tumors of the supratentorial compartment (cPNET), pineoblastomas, and atypical teratoid/rhabdoid tumors (AT/RT). After the general PNET concept coined by the neuropathologist LB Rorke [10] it is now recognized that these tumors former uniformly called PNET are subdivided according to their localization [11]. The reason for this strategy among others is that they show differing results after treatment.

© Springer International Publishing Switzerland 2017
M. Warmuth-Metz, *Imaging and Diagnosis in Pediatric Brain Tumor Studies*,
DOI 10.1007/978-3-319-42503-0_3

3.2.1 Medulloblastoma

MBs are the most frequent malignant tumors of childhood. They grow in the cerebellum. Meanwhile five different histological and four genetic variants [12] of this tumor are known and characterized by differences in prognosis, morphology and localization (Table 3.1). All MBs are highly cellular tumors. High cell density is translated into a low T2-signal and a restricted diffusion leading to a high signal on diffusion images and a dark presentation on an ADC map (acquired diffusion coefficient) [13]. On CT before contrast enhancement the solid parts of the tumors are mostly hyperdense [14] compared to the cerebellar cortex (Fig. 3.1). Of course necroses or rare cysts do not show high CT density. In our far more than 100 CTs of MBs we did not encounter a single tumor showing hypodense CT-values in the solid parts of the tumor.

3.2.1.1   MB with Extensive Nodularity (See Table 3.1)

Young children (all below 3 years of age in our database with a mean age of 1 year) are the typical age group for MBs with extensive nodularity (MBEN). It is a subtype of the desmoplastic nodular variant. MBENs bear a much better prognosis with adequate treatment and can be cured with chemotherapy even if they present with an otherwise bad prognostic sign of a meningeal dissemination [15]. They may show rare recurrences, which usually can be salvaged by additional treatment. Interestingly MBEN are very dark on ADC or T2-weighted images suggesting a high cell density (Fig. 3.2a). They often contain cysts and an intense tubular enhancement (Fig. 3.2b) that was also described as grape-like [15]. In an evaluation of 470 MB in our database all 15 MBEN showed complete and intense enhancement and 11 of the 15 tumors showed the typical enhancement pattern mentioned above. Interestingly MBEN are the MBs with the largest perifocal edema. All other varieties show no or little edema. This result underlines that a larger edema cannot be considered as a general sign of a more malignant tumor.

Table 3.1 MB histological variants

Subtype	Age at diagnosis (median/ range)	Localization midline/ hemisphere (in %)	Contrast enhancement >50% volume (in %)	Meningeal dissemination at diagnosis (in %)	Tumor size (volume in ml)
CMB $n=356$	7 (1–21)	97/3	61	14	32
DMB $n=75$	7 (1–19)	72/28	84	8	38
MBEN $n=15$	1 (0–3)	93/7	100	7	60
AMB $n=12$	6 (2–16)	92/8	92	8	26
LCMB $n=7$	7 (2–14)	100/0	86	71	15

Demographic and imaging results of 465 MB patients in the database of the reference center for Neuroradiology of the HIT-Studies

Abbreviations: *MB* medulloblastoma, *CMB* classic MB, *DMB* desmoplastic MB, *MBEN* MB with extensive nodularity, *AMB* anaplastic MB, *LCMB* large cell MB

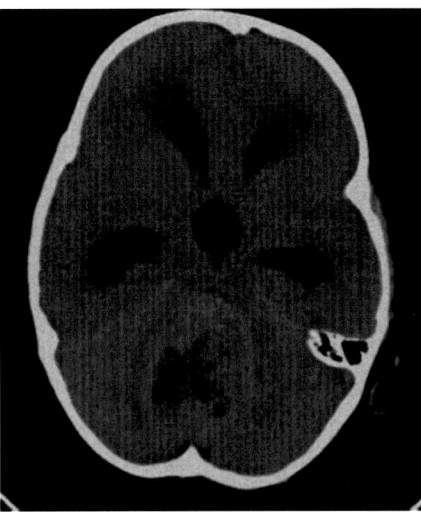

Fig. 3.1 Classic medulloblastoma: a CT before contrast shows a tumor in the fourth ventricle with obstructive hydrocephalus. The solid parts of the tumor are hyperdense compared to the gray matter of the cerebellum signifying high cellularity. Central necrotic parts are hypodense and characteristically no significant edema is surrounding the tumor. The high density excludes a low-grade glioma. However, also an ependymoma could be possible in this case

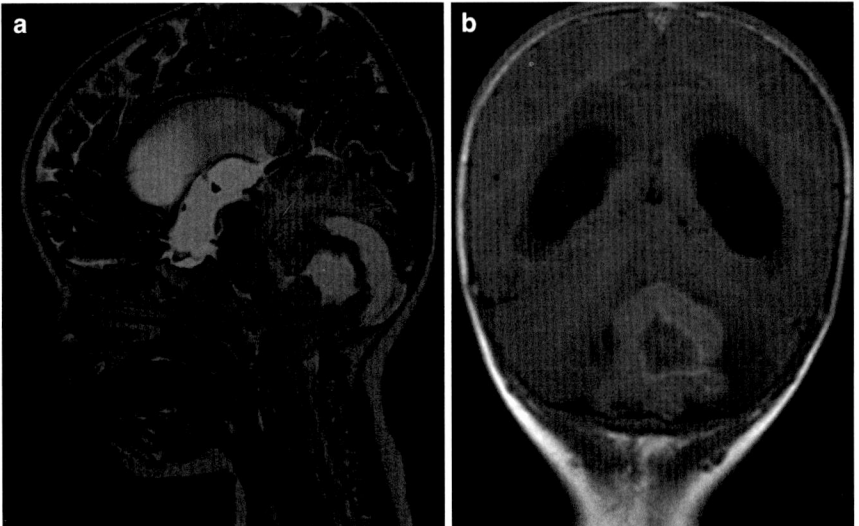

Fig. 3.2 (**a**) Sagittal T2-w MRI: In a child aged 18 months a tumor in the cerebellar posterior midline shows very low T2-signal in his solid areas and a large perifocal edema. Age, localization, T2-signal, and amount of perifocal edema are very characteristic of an MBEN. (**b**) Coronal enhanced T1-w sequence: The solid portion of an MBEN in another young child shows an intense and band-like enhancement

3.2.1.2 Desmoplastic-Nodular MB (See Table 3.1)

The desmoplastic-nodular MBs peak at two different ages [16]. They affect young children and have been shown to have a much better prognosis than all the remaining subtypes in young children with the exception of MBEN. The second age peak lies in the second decade or even older ages. Also these tumors are usually more benign than, e.g., classic MBs. Desmoplastic-nodular MBs enhance intensely and most frequently entirely (Fig. 3.3a, b) and a nodular enhancement pattern resembling the histopathological appearance may be seen. Desmoplastic-nodular MB in our database and all the other subtypes had their typical peak age between 5 and 9 years.

3.2.1.3 Anaplastic and Large Cell MB (See Table 3.1)

These two MB variants have been grouped together before the WHO classification published in 2007 and have been separated thereafter [17]. They are quite rare. Anaplastic MBs do not seem to behave as bad concerning prognosis as their name pretends [18]. In our 470 MB we did not find very specific imaging features that might allow a probable diagnosis by imaging in this variant. However, large-cell MBs are usually prognostically grave [18] and are metastatic in the cerebrospinal fluid (CSF) in up to 70 % already at diagnosis. The tumors are small at diagnosis and contrast enhancement is variable (Fig. 3.4). In large cell MB probably the clinical complaints by the meningeal dissemination lead to the diagnosis and not so frequently the symptoms of the tumor itself.

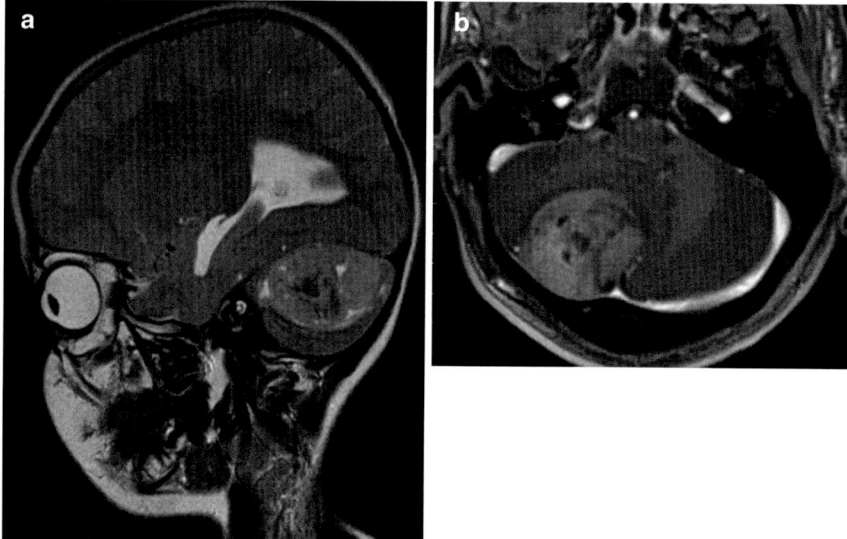

Fig. 3.3 (a) Parasagittal T2-weighted MRI in a young child with a desmoplastic-nodular MB. The nodular aspect of the solid tumor in the cerebellar hemisphere and the vicinity to the superficial structures is characteristic for desmoplastic nodular MBs. (b) In another patient, a young adult, the typical position superficially in the right cerebellar hemisphere is fitting to a desmoplastic nodular subtype of MB

3.2.1.4 Classic MB (See Table 3.1)

Classic MBs are the most frequent MB (356 out of 465 MB). They rather frequently show a diminished or no contrast uptake (10 % in our database) (Table 3.2) compared to the regularly and mostly completely enhancing other subtypes (Fig. 3.5a). Only about 40 % are enhancing entirely.

3.2.1.5 Typical Localization of the MB Variants

The most frequent classic subtype is usually localized within the cerebellar dorsal midline (Fig. 3.5b). Only 3 % of our 356 classic MB were found outside the midline

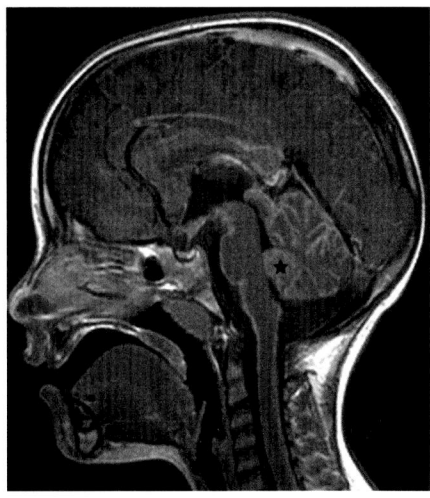

Fig. 3.4 The sagittal enhanced T1-w sequence shows a small large-cell MB (*asterisk*) and an impressive laminar and nodular dissemination in the cranial and spinal CSF

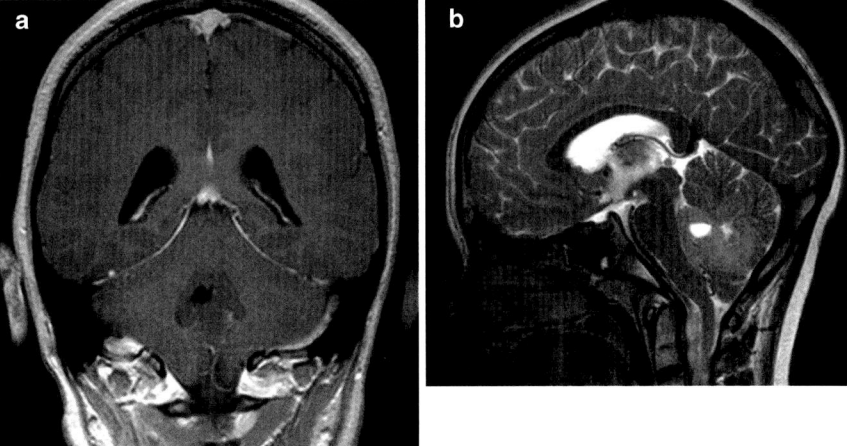

Fig. 3.5 (**a**) On a coronal enhanced T1-weighted MRI, the classic MB does not show any enhancement. Little or no enhancement is most frequent in the classic subtype. (**b**) A midline position in the cerebellar vermis is characteristic for most MBs and the classic subtype in special (same patient as in Fig. 3.5a)

Fig. 3.6 T2-weighted axial MRI
showing a WNT-type medulloblastoma
in a quite typical lateral position in the
cerebellopontine angle

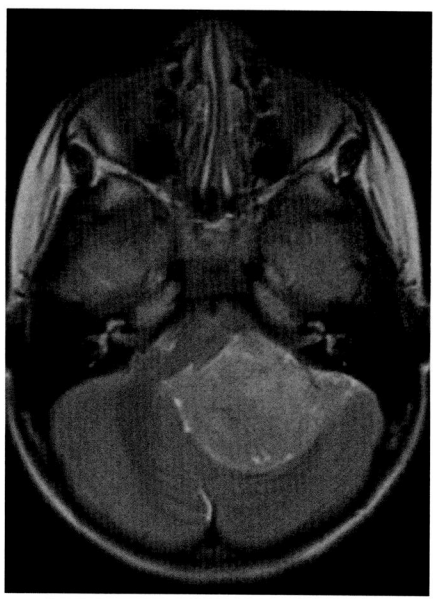

in the hemispheres and possibly could also represent brainstem PNET, because histologically PNET and MB look the same and can only be allocated by their respective localization. This differential diagnosis is important as brainstem PNET are prognostically worse due to the inherent inability to resect them substantially.

In the second most frequent histological subtype the desmoplastic-nodular type the typical localization within the superficial parts of the cerebellar hemisphere (Fig. 3.3a, b) is predominantly found in teenagers and young (or rarely older) adults [19]. An infiltration of dural structures or even a crossing of the tentorium is not unusual [20]. This histological subtype in young children is much more often localized in the vermis alike the classic type [21]. Also MBEN are mainly found a midline position [22].

The anaplastic and large-cell MBs are also frequently found in the midline.

Not yet completely scientifically evaluated also genetic subtypes may have certain predominant localizations. It has recently been found that three out of four of the wingless pathway activated (WNT) MBs were localized in an off-midline position near the lateral brain stem with extension into the cerebellopontine (CP) angle [23] mimicking ependymomas, which are frequent in this area. In our own 290 genetically classified MB this was the case in 50 % of 18 WNT MBs (Fig. 3.6).

3.2.1.6   Differential Diagnosis (See Table 3.3)

Ependymomas in the posterior fossa are highly cellular tumors and cannot be differentiated from MB by T2- and ADC-brightness or CT-density. The internal structure with cyst-like necrotic areas, the localization in the lower fourth ventricle, and near to the ependymal layer in the cerebellopontine angle, and the growth behavior (plastic growth) may be the differentiating clue. For details please see Sect. 3.3.

Table 3.2 Decision tree for the probable diagnosis of a suprasellar tumor in a child

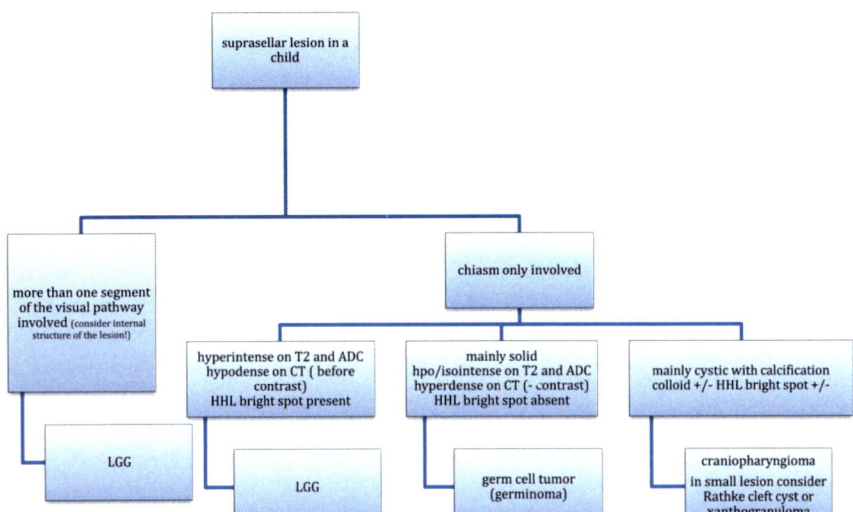

Pilocytic astrocytomas are the most frequent low-grade tumors in children at all, and in the posterior fossa they have a predilection site. They histologically show a low cellularity and therefore display a very bright T2-signal. They do not show restricted but increased diffusion and are hypodense in their solid parts on CT. Enhancement is frequent but variable and does not allow a differential diagnosis. See Sect. 3.2.1.

In case of a very young child below 6 or 12 months of age you should also think of an AT/RT. Bleeding residues, an off midline position and peripheral cysts as well as a peculiar enhancement pattern are rather intriguing. See Sect. 3.1.3.

Hemangioblastomas are tumors that usually do not affect very young children. The peak incidence is in the second decade as well as for syndromal hemangioblastomas in von Hippel-Lindau syndrome as also sporadic ones [24]. Details are covered in the Sect. 3.2.1.

Choroid plexus papillomas can arise everywhere where plexus is found. They usually show a high CT-density and low T2-signal. The correct diagnosis can be suspected, if a multinodular smooth surface (cauliflower-like aspect) and a strong enhancement resembling a normal choroid plexus are seen. Many patients do not show specific symptoms, and these tumors can be found incidentally. They tend to bloc the CSF pathways and can lead to clinical symptoms associated to hydrocephalus. More aggressive choroid tumors are atypical plexus papillomas (WHO grade II) and plexus carcinomas (WHO grade III). The morphological differences on neuroimaging may not be obvious between these entities. Of course carcinomas tend to show signs of infiltration into the brain while papillomas are usually sharply margined and confined to the ventricular lumen. Carcinomas are more frequently inhomogenous and large tumors. A leptomeningeal dissemination may be seen in all three variants and does not exclude a grade I papilloma.

Plexus carcinomas can very well resemble AT/RTs on imaging. Interestingly common features in immunohistochemistry between these two entities have been described [25].

3.2.2 Central Nervous System Primitive Neuroectodermal Tumors (CNS PNET changed to ETMR in the new WHO classification)

CNS PNETs arise in the cerebral hemispheres, the brain stem, and the spinal cord [26] of children and mainly young adults. A variant of this clinically very aggressive entity according to a specific differentiation are cerebral neuroblastomas or ganglio-neuroblastomas, medulloepitheliomas, and ependymoblastomas. On imaging we see highly cellular tumors with a low T2 and restricted diffusion (Fig. 3.7a–c). Contrast enhancement is variable but more frequently sparse than intense or complete (Fig. 3.7d). It is often missing completely. Perifocal edema is mostly minor or absent (Fig. 3.7e), and in contradiction to a fast growth and malignant behavior the tumor seems to be surrounded by a capsule and usually is on imaging well delineated from the surrounding brain [27]. Like MB also CNS PNET are prone to tumor dissemination in the leptomeninges prompting an MRI evaluation of the complete cranial and spinal CSF space.

3.2.3 Atypical Teratoid/Rhabdoid Tumor (AT/RT)

AT/RTs are highly malignant tumors affecting young children. Meanwhile they are considered the most frequent malignant brain tumors within the first 6 months of age [28, 29]. They are closely linked to rhabdoid tumors of the kidneys as well on histology as also genetic findings and may be found in familial rhabdoid tumor predisposition syndrome [30, 31]. AT/RTs are restricted to the CNS and supra- or infratentorial localization is varying with age. Older children or rarely adults more frequently develop supratentorial tumors [32]. AT/RTs may also arise in the spinal cord [33, 34] and are then not distinguishable from other cord tumors.

In the brain it is rather the combination of multiple features than one single characteristic on imaging that can help to find the likely diagnosis. Like all tumors with increased cell density, the solid parts are very hypointense on T2-weighted MRI and

Fig. 3.7 T2-weighted axial (**a**) and sagittal (**e**) MRI, diffusion-weighted MRI (**b**) and ADC (**c**) and T1-weighted image after contrast enhancement (**d**) of different children with a cPNET. It is characteristic that cPNETs are sharply delineated without perifocal edema. The high cell density is reflected by a restricted diffusion and thus a dark ADC. Contrast enhancement is frequently little or missing

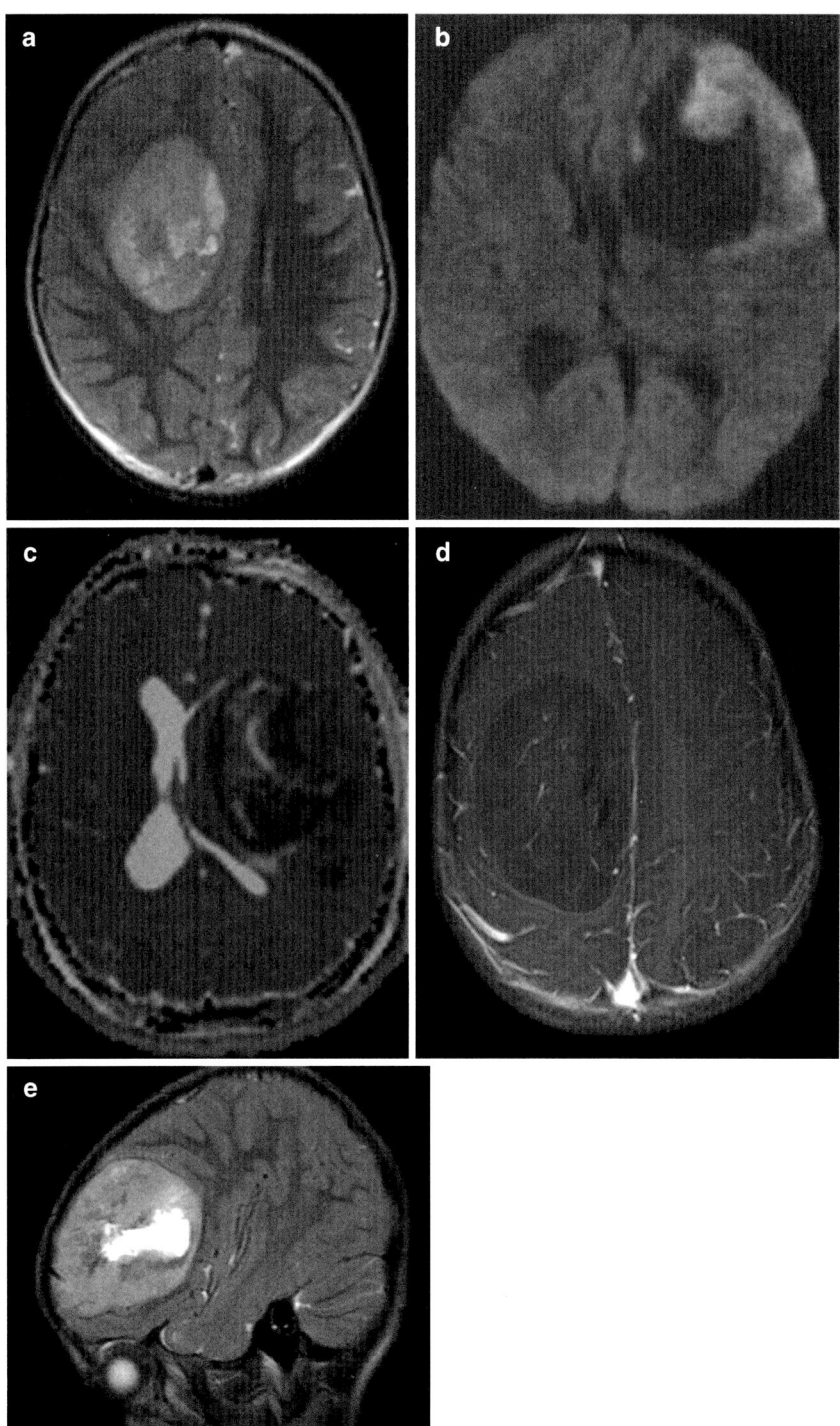

show a severely restricted diffusion on ADC (Fig. 3.8a). Being often hemorrhagic on macroscopic inspection, the deposition of blood products like hemosiderin or methemoglobin is quite characteristic (Fig. 3.8b). Peripheral cysts placed in between the surface of the tumor and the normal brain have been described frequently [32, 35] (Fig. 3.8c). Usually the borders are surrounded by a varying amount of perifocal edema. The amount of the perifocal edema can be used for the differentiation to PNETs. An astonishingly high percentage of bone destruction of the vault or skull base has been found, which is an extremely unusual feature in other primary CNS tumors [36]. In a number of patients, a characteristic band-like wavy pattern of contrast enhancement surrounding a more or less large central necrotic area is visible [32, 35] (Fig. 3.8d). Together with a young age these imaging characteristics can be used in the differential diagnosis of an AT/RT.

3.3 Glial Tumors

3.3.1 Astrocytomas

Low-grade astrocytomas and among those the main representative of circumscribed astrocytomas, the juvenile pilocytic astrocytoma, are the most frequent brain tumors in children and young adults [37]. More often the origin is the cerebellum followed by the supratentorial midline, synonym for the surroundings of the third ventricle, the chiasm and hypothalamus, and other parts of the visual pathway [38]. However, pilocytic astrocytomas may grow anywhere in the CNS and are the most frequent tumors of the spinal cord in children, while in adults ependymomas of the spinal cord are predominant [39]. A typical combination of an enhancing nodule and cystic tumor parts (Fig. 3.9a) has been described as characteristic imaging feature [40]. However, purely solid or regularly enhancing tumors are not rare (Fig. 3.9b, c) and might lead to a misclassification as possible high-grade tumor. This can be avoided easily, if the distinctive low cellularity of the tumor is respected. The low cellular density is correlated to a bright intensity on T2-weighted MRI (Fig. 3.9d) and a high ADC (Fig. 3.9e) value without any suspicion of restricted diffusion in the solid parts of the tumor. The only pitfall may be blood product deposition (Fig. 3.9f) or calcification within the tumor that might render this discriminating feature useless by possibly lowering the T2-signal [41] and the ADC as well. A low density of solid tumor on unenhanced CT is a regular finding in noncalcified low-grade gliomas and can be used as a differential diagnostic tool (Fig. 3.9g). Interestingly we only found hyperdense CT-values in LGGs in patients with NF1 without knowing why they differ from sporadic tumors. Germ cell tumors, e.g., exhibit iso- but mainly hyperdense values.

In the spinal cord no differentiation between the various histologies is possible and the suspicion of a pilocytic astrocytoma is only based on the age of the affected patient and not on imaging characteristics. In ependymomas, rarely hemosiderin deposits are diagnostic either as leptomeningeal hemosiderosis (Fig. 3.10) or as hemosiderin caps at the upper and lower borders of the tumor [42–44].

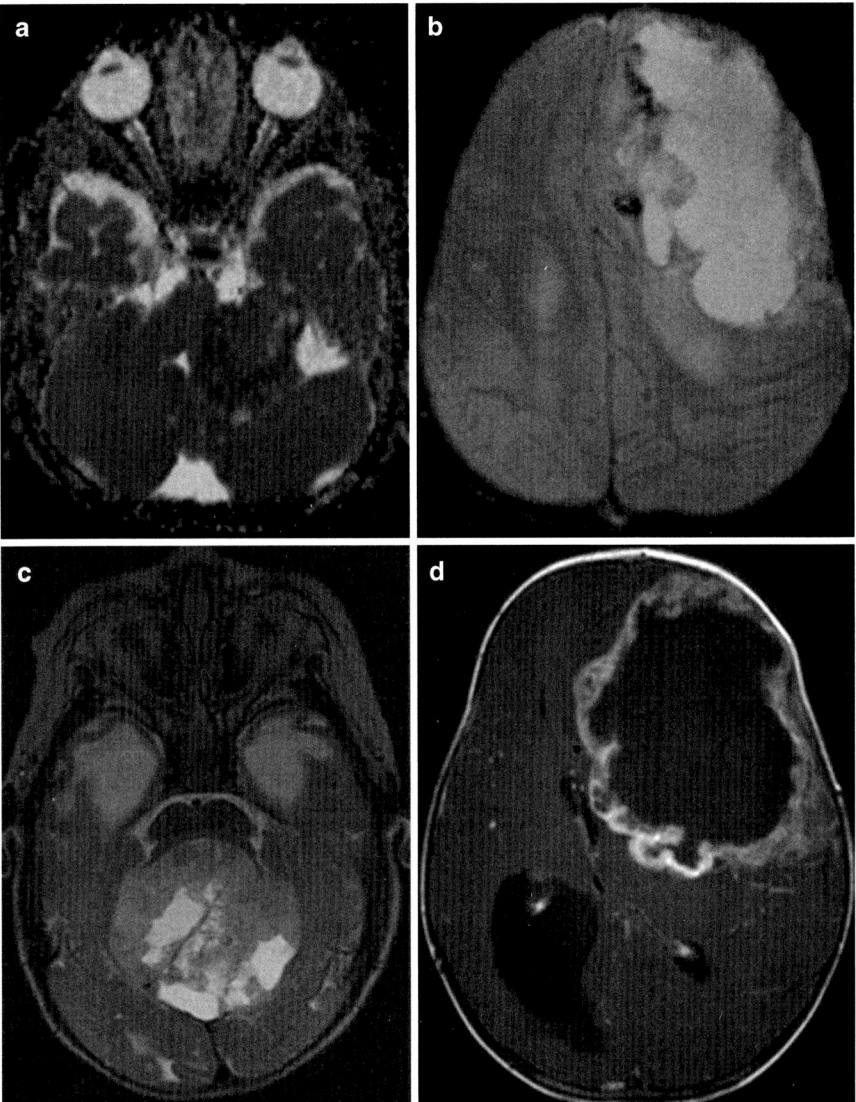

Fig. 3.8 Axial diffusion-weighted MRI (**a**), iron-sensitive T2*-image (**b**), T2-weighted image (**c**), and postcontrast T1-weighted MRI (**d**). Same patient on (**b**) and (**d**). AT/RTs are highly cellular tumors with a very dark ADC (**a**). A midline position (**c**) in the posterior fossa is less frequent than an off-midline growth. Characteristic features are residues of bleeding (**b**) and a rather peculiar pattern of a band-like enhancement surrounding a central necrosis and the existence of peripheral cyst-like lesions (**c**)

3.3.1.1 Visual Pathway Gliomas

About 20 % of children with neurofibromatosis type I (NF1) or von Recklinghausen's disease develop visual pathway gliomas [45]. NF I is a phacomatosis with various defects in the tumor suppressor gene located on the long arm of chromosome 17 [46].

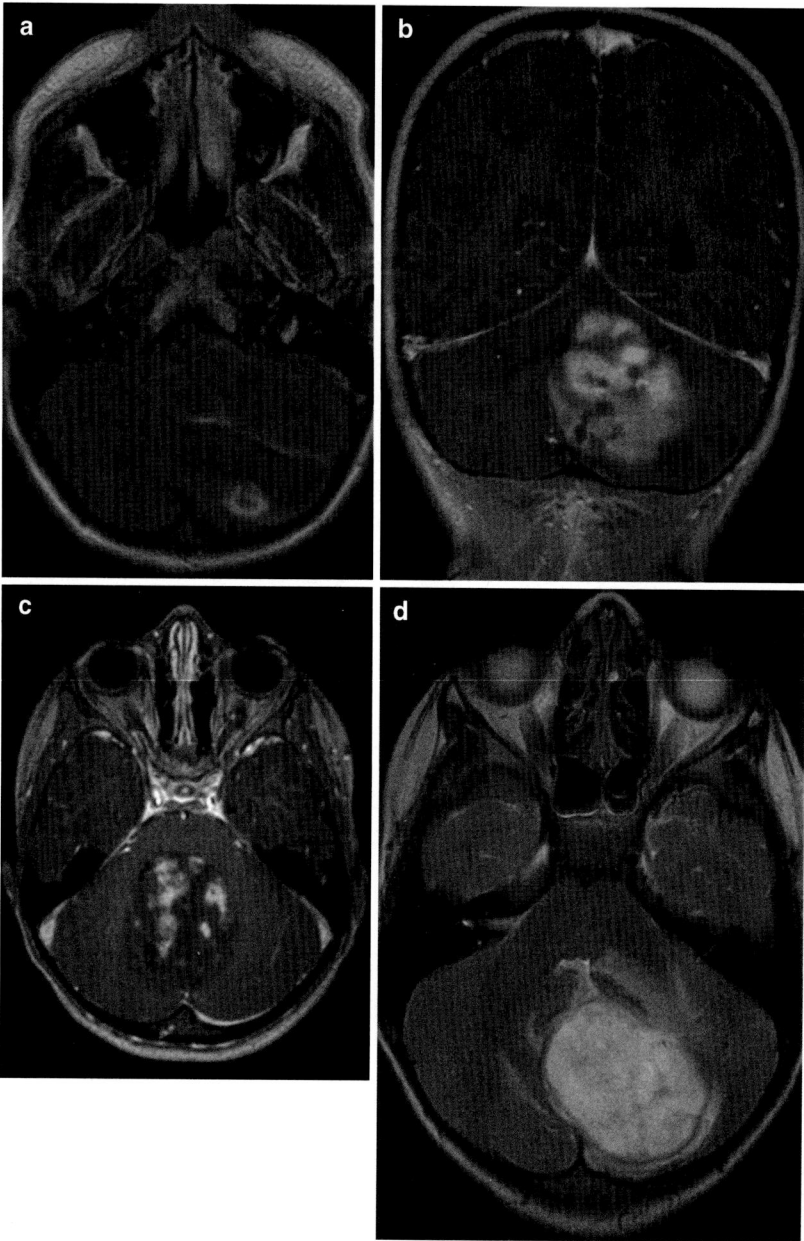

Fig. 3.9 (a–c) Axial (**a**, **c**) and coronal (**b**) T1-weighted postcontrast MRIs of different patients. The pathognomic pattern of a nidus and a cyst (**a**) is not unique. Enhancement may be complete with characteristic smooth margins (**b**) or incomplete and irregular (**c**) mimicking a high-grade glioma. Axial T2-weighted (**d**) and ADC (**e**) images of different children showing the bright signal signifying a low cell density and facilitated diffusion. Pilocytic astrocytomas have pathologic vessels and therefore iron deposition and increased vessel density on SWI (**f**) (pilocytic astrocytoma in the mediobasal right temporal lobe) must not be considered as a sign of a higher malignancy grade as in adult high-grade gliomas. Low cell density is affecting the density values of unenhanced CT (**g**) leading to mainly hypodense solid components

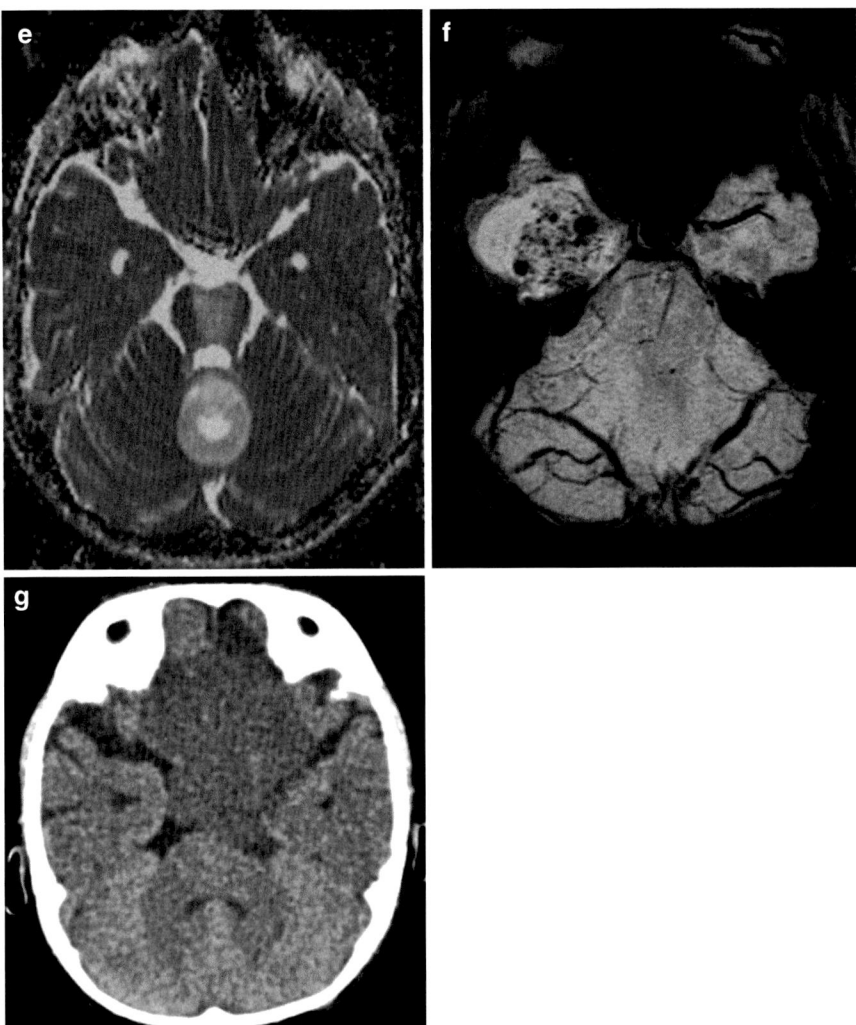

Fig. 3.9 (continued)

The incidence of CNS tumors and among those especially tumors of the visual pathway is increased. The visual pathway consists of several segments that have been classified according to Dodge in three parts [47]. Dodge I is tumor in the optic nerve uni- or bilaterally (Fig. 3.11a). The second part is the optic chiasm where sporadic, non-NF1-associated, gliomas are found most frequently. The affection of the chiasm with or without the optic nerves is called Dodge II (Fig. 3.11b). Dodge III is reserved for tumors of the optic tracts or radiation either with or without a participation of the anterior visual pathway [48] (Fig. 3.11c). Visual pathway gliomas in NF1 are predominantly diffuse tumors occupying long distances of the visual pathway and tumors of the posterior pathway. Tumors in the posterior pathway are more frequently associated with severe problems of vision and blindness. This traditional classification is quite approximate and does not allow a detailed anatomically based analysis of the

Fig. 3.10 Sagittal T2-weighted MRI
in a young adult patient with a
lumbosacral ependymoma and an
extensive leptomeningeal hemosiderin
deposition, which is rare but
pathognomonic for this histology

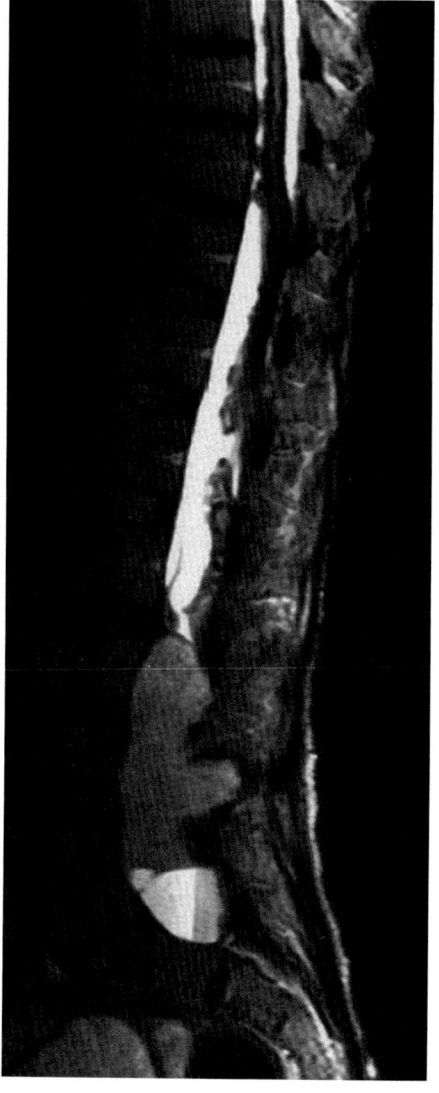

affected parts of the pathway. Oncologists and radiologists from Padua, Leeds, Augsburg and Nottingham (PLAN) have settled out to find a more refined classification, the so-called PLAN system [49], by classifying the tumors of a number of children from these four hospitals. It is a quite detailed system, introduced to allow risk evaluation especially for disturbances of vision. The main problem of the PLAN classification is that size changes of the tumor do necessarily lead to an involvement of a different part of the pathway and are thus not reflected by this system. As a consequence, the tumor might grow considerably and the PLAN stage does not change. However, a more common use of the PLAN classification is needed to decide on the usefulness for the patients and treatment decisions because vision is the main criterion of outcome for children with visual pathway tumors. Nearly all tumors affecting more

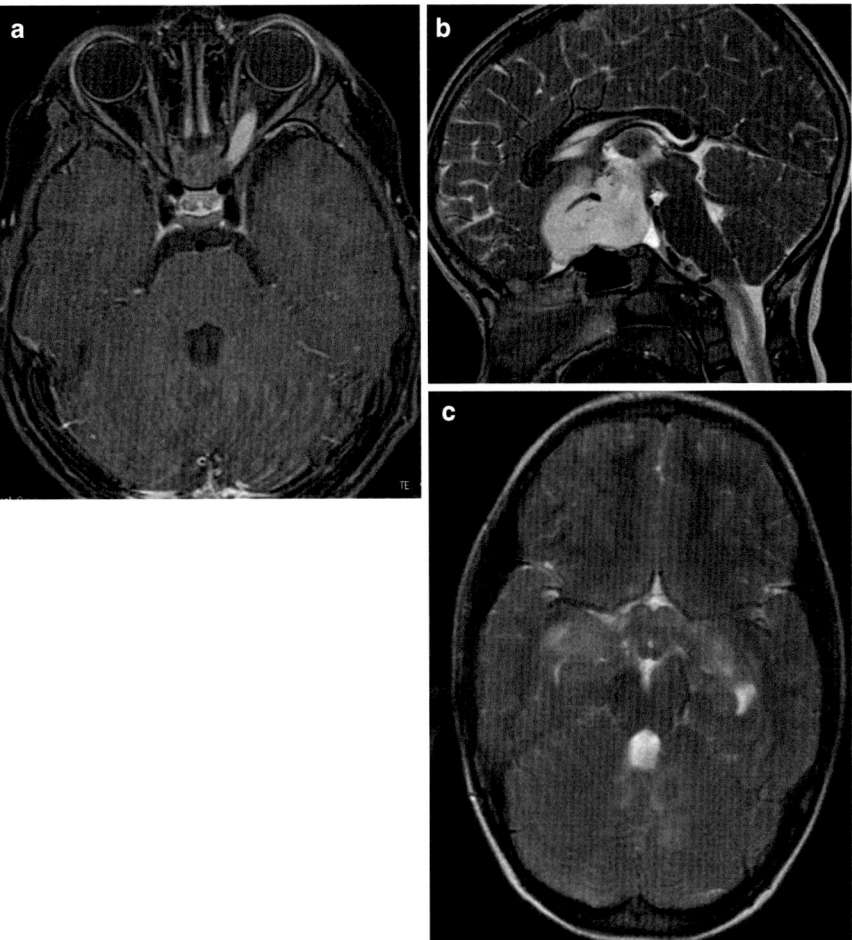

Fig. 3.11 Visual pathway gliomas in different children. In Dodge I (**a**, axial T1-weighted MRI after contrast) only one or both optic nerves are affected. In (**a**) the left optic nerve shows enhancement and slight thickening. The Dodge stage II is characterized by a glioma in the chiasmatic-hypothalamic region as seen on the sagittal T2-weighted MRI (**b**) with an extension into the subfrontal region. If the tracts and radiation are involved as seen on the T2-weighted MRI of a patient with NF-1 (**c**) this corresponds to Dodge III. Mark the involvement of the chiasm and hypothalamus and the multiple T2-signal increases in the cerebellar white matter characteristic in middle aged children with NF-1

than one part of the visual pathway in children are low-grade gliomas (LGG) (astrocytomas WHO grade I or II and gangliogliomas WHO grade I). In this context, only one situation might create differential diagnostic problems. A compression of the chiasm by any kind of lesion may lead to an edema in the optic tracts (Fig. 3.12a, b). This phenomenon was first described in craniopharyngiomas [50] but may happen in any kind of tumor like, e.g., in germ cell tumors or even in metastases in adults [51]. The clue to a correct classification is to consider and compare the internal structure of the chiasmatic and tract lesions. If they differ then a reactive edema of the tracts due to some other tumor in the chiasm is very likely.

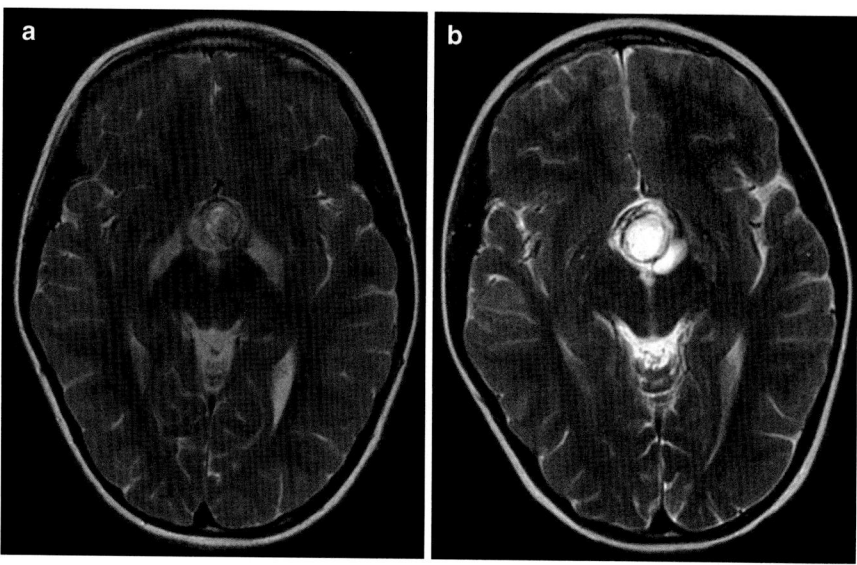

Fig. 3.12 If more than one segment of the visual pathway are affected by a lesion this is virtually nearly always a glioma. A pitfall, however, is the development of a tract edema in chiasmatic tumors like, e.g., craniopharyngiomas and all kinds of usually larger and compressive other tumors. To avoid this false diagnosis you have to evaluate the internal structure of lesions in the chiasm and the tracts. On the T2-weighted axial MRI there is a clear difference between the lesion in the chiasm, a germ cell tumor, and the hypersignal in the tracts at diagnosis (**a**). After treatment the mass lesion has diminished and a control MRI after 3 months (**b**) shows that the edema on the right hand side has vanished and is markedly reduced on the left hand side

3.3.1.2 Differential Diagnosis of Suprasellar and Visual Pathway Lesions

Extremely rare in children are high-grade gliomas (anaplastic astrocytomas or GBM) [52] of the visual pathway. The few cases in our patients were predominant in the chiasm and visually not distinguishable from LGG. Inflammation like sarcoidosis affecting more than one part of the visual pathway [53] has been published in adults and occasionally in adolescents [54] as an accepted differential diagnostic option to diffuse visual pathway gliomas. Sarcoidosis is at least in my experience not found in younger children, who mainly bear gliomas of the visual pathway. Perhaps our patients represent a selection in this respect. If the lesion is confined to only one segment of the pathway like the chiasm, plenty of different tumors might be possible and an accurate differentiation is needed. Here again the high T2- and ADC-signal as a sign of low cellular density in LGG plays an important role. Another crucial sign is the preservation of the normal posterior pituitary lobe (PPL) bright spot (Fig. 3.13a). The bright spot correlates to a collection of vasopressin in the PPL [55]. The loss of the bright PPL signal is frequently accompanied clinically by diabetes insipidus [56]. The bright spot is best seen on T1-weighted sequences

Table 3.3 Decision tree for the probable diagnosis of tumors in the posterior fossa in a child

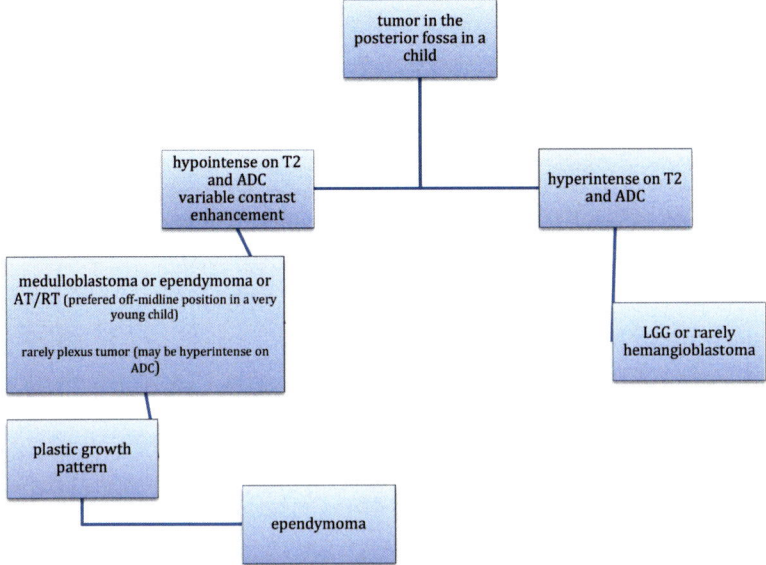

before the application of contrast medium and indicates a normal function of the connection between hypothalamus and PPL. T1-weighted sequences with fatsupression technique may be useful for an easier detection of the bright spot because the reliable distinction on a standard T1-image between the normal PPL bright spot and fat in the sella or around the pituitary gland can be hard or impossible. The best way to identify the PPL bright spot is on thin sagittal T1-weighted images (SL, e.g., 2–3 mm). We prefer spin echo (SE) or turbo spin echo (TSE) images by far compared, e.g., to MPR sequences. While the PPL bright spot is practically always present in LGGs affecting the suprasellar region, it is nearly regularly missing in germ cell tumors of the same region [57] (Fig. 3.13b). It may be preserved or missing in craniopharyngiomas depending on their size and individual location (Fig. 3.13c, d). Usually the size of the pituitary gland is diminished in craniopharyngiomas (Fig. 3.13d) and germ cell tumors, which is frequently accompanied by an insufficiency of the pituitary function [58]. Important differential diagnostic signs are the presence of calcifications or colloid in adamantinous craniopharyngiomas of childhood, which are characteristically predominantly cystic tumors. Contrary to adults affected by craniopharyngiomas, the adamantinous type of histology is by far the most frequent type. Adults usually bear papillary craniopharyngiomas that are more solid and homogeneous tumors without calcifications [59]. Larger cysts are missing in germinomas, the most frequent germ cell tumor in adolescents and young adults. If cysts and an inhomogeneous internal structure are seen in a germ cell tumor, this is rather a sign of a mixed or secreting germ cell tumor because the teratoma parts exhibit a more inhomogeneous structure [60, 61].

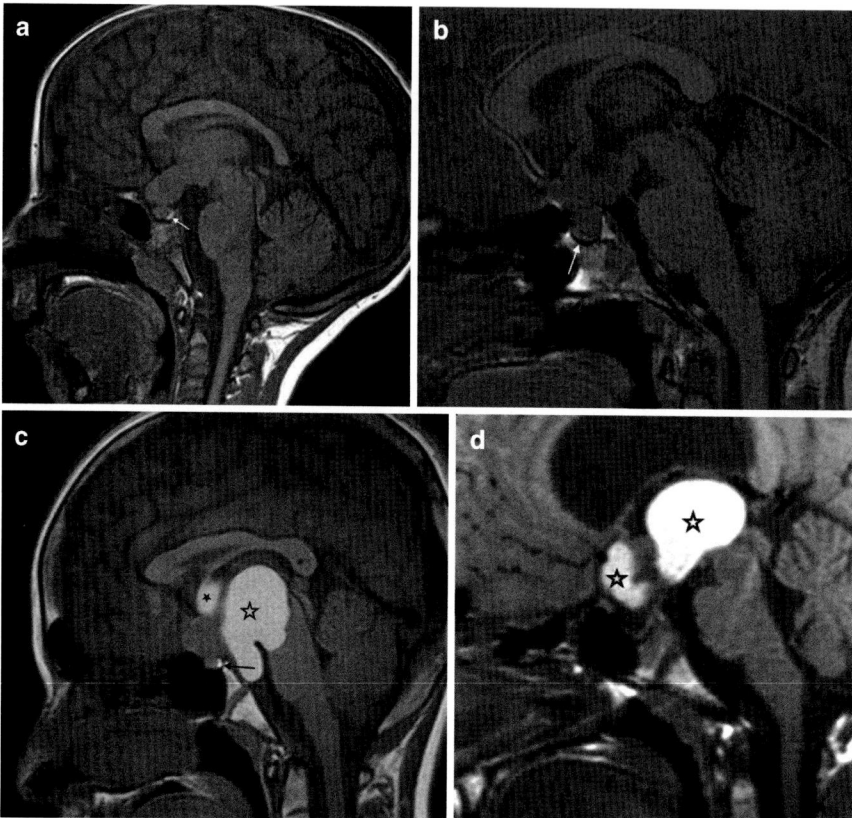

Fig. 3.13 Diagnostic significance of the bright pituitary spot on unenhanced T1-weighted MRI. In LGGs (**a**) virtually always the physiological hyperintensity of the posterior pituitary lobe (*arrow*) is present, while this bright spot is very frequently missing in suprasellar germ cell tumors (**b**). Note the compressed pituitary gland (*arrow*) below the tumor extending into the third ventricle. In craniopharyngiomas (**c**, **d**) the behavior of the bright spot is not predictable and depends on the site and size of the tumor. In (**c**) it is present despite a large tumor with colloid filled cysts (*asterisk*). In (**d**) it is absent. Note the flat and very small pituitary gland

3.3.2   Gliomas of Higher Grades (HGG)

Comparable to gliomas of higher grades of malignancies in adults, HGG in children tend to show more indistinct margins, larger perifocal edema, and areas of higher cell density or necrosis. However, a differentiation between entities or grades is not possible with a reasonable certainty on the basis of imaging alone in an individual patient. So the suspicion of a high-grade glioma may be raised but a definite diagnosis is usually not possible by MRI (or CT) (Fig. 3.14a–d).

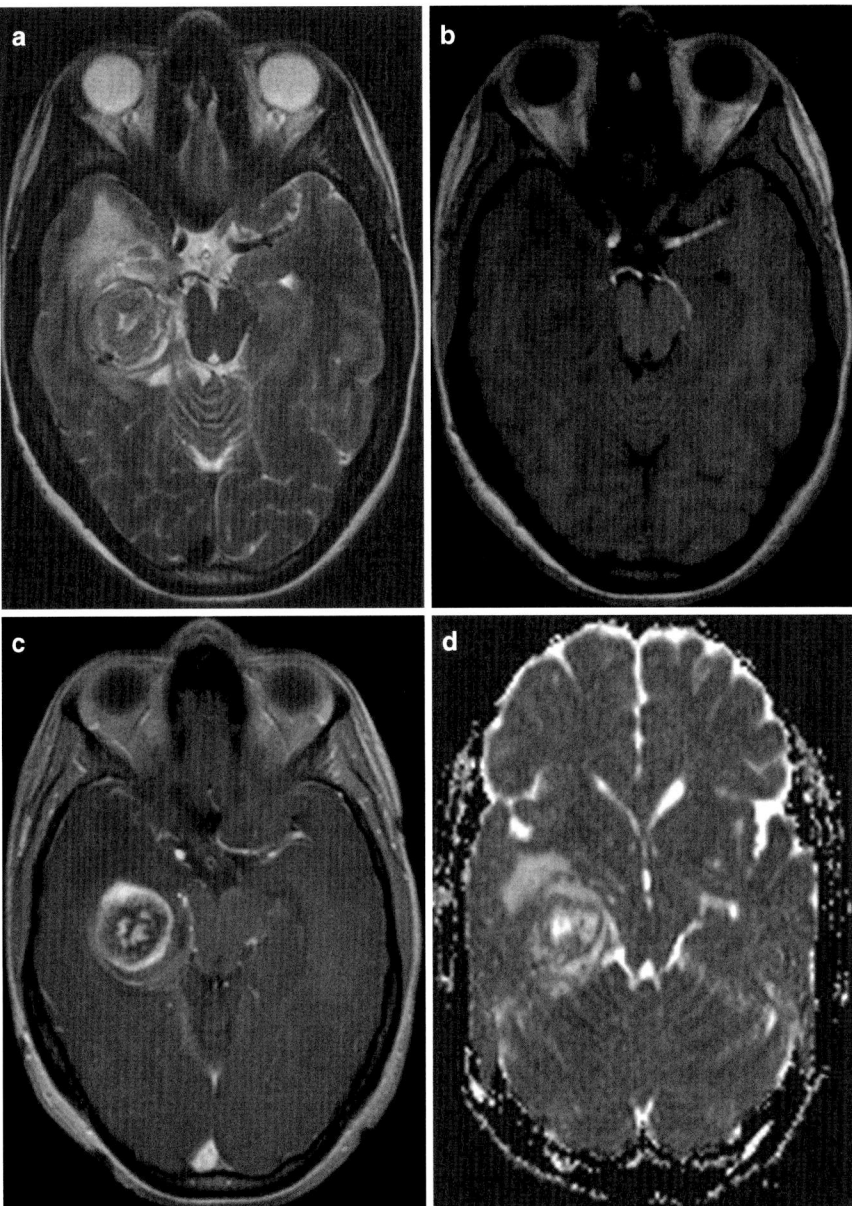

Fig. 3.14 In high-grade gliomas the prediction of tumor type and WHO grade is much less precise. General but rather nonprecise predictors of a high WHO-grade are: inhomogeneous tumor with larger perifocal edema and indistinct margins (**a,** T2-weighted axial MRI). Blood product deposition like met-hemoglobin on T1-weighted MRI before contrast (**b**). Irregular, increasing enhancement after contrast medium application (**c**). Areas with a higher cell density than in low-grade gliomas (**d**: ADC)

3.3.2.1   Gliomatosis Cerebri (omitted acc. to the new WHO-classification)

According to the WHO classification 2007, gliomatosis cerebri is defined as a diffuse growth of a glioma grade II–IV within more than two cerebral lobes [62] (Fig. 3.15a). The central parts of the brain like basal ganglia or thalami may be involved or not and growth into the infratentorial compartment or even the spinal cord may be present or not (Fig. 3.15b). As a consequence this definition only applies to supratentorial tumors. Usually the mass effect is not predominant and contrast enhancement like in DIPG may signify higher grades but is not essential for the diagnosis (Fig. 3.15c) because also on biopsy vascular hyperplasia is usually missing [63]. Frequently, inflammation like encephalitis is the initial suspicion because many patients develop a seizure as the first symptom. These tumors are never completely resectable and prognosis is therefore grave like in other diffuse gliomas depending on age, Karnofsky performance status, and WHO grade of the gliomatosis. Comparable to gliomatosis cerebri, the prognosis of multifocal gliomas (Fig. 3.15d–f) is grave because multifocal diffuse lesions are usually also not resectable. Contrary to embryonal tumors like MBs, gliomas may grow in separate parts of the brain parenchyma either synchronously or during progression [64, 65].

3.3.2.2   Brain Stem Gliomas

Depending on their localization, the WHO grade and prognosis of brain stem gliomas differ considerably. The following description of individual entities is ordered according to the tumor site.

3.3.2.3   Cerebral Peduncles

The most frequent gliomas in this localization in children are low-grade gliomas, predominantly pilocytic astrocytomas [66–68] (Fig. 3.16a–d). They are usually sharply demarcated and may extend as well into the basal ganglia as downwards into the pons. It is of utmost importance to respect the main mass of the tumor and its localization in the brain stem to discriminate these gliomas from the typical diffuse intrinsic pontine gliomas. Symptomatic tumors in the cerebral peduncles are usually decompressed by neurosurgery and therefore a histological clarification is the regular consequence.

3.3.2.4   Tectal Plate Gliomas

Tectal plate gliomas belong frequently to the group of presumably low-grade gliomas [68], although a histological clarification is usually not performed in the majority of uncomplicated cases. They become symptomatic not by regional disturbances

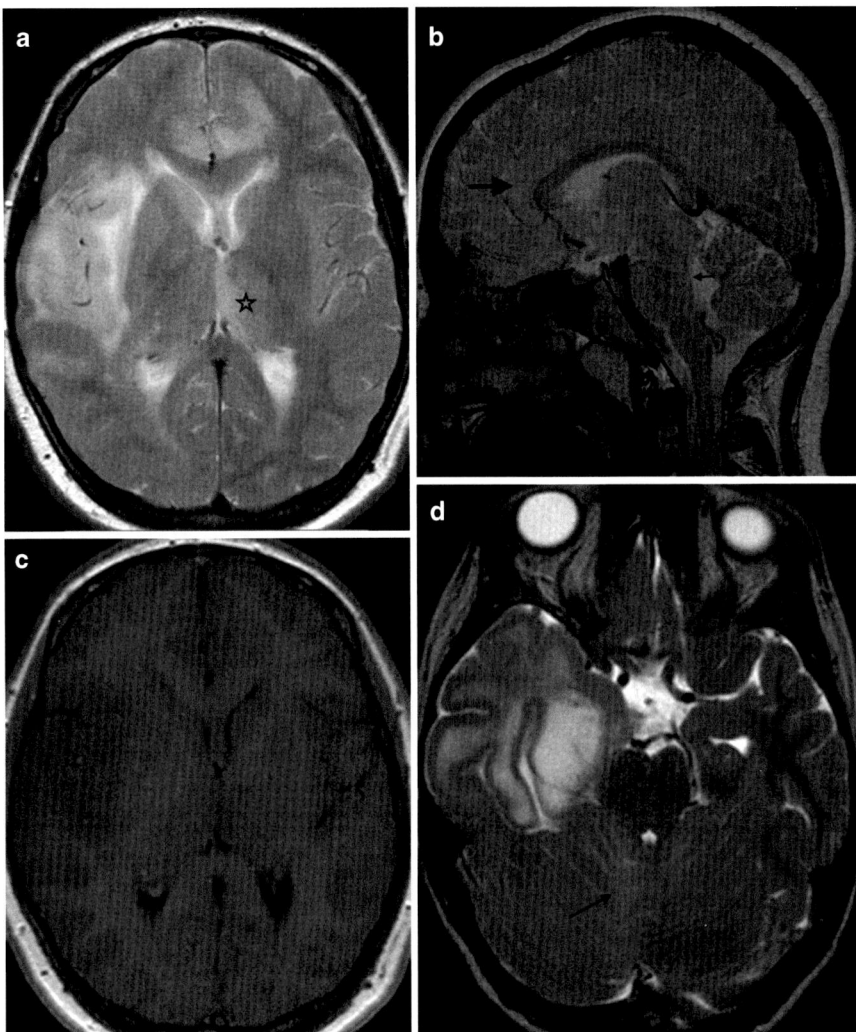

Fig. 3.15 (**a–f**) Gliomatosis cerebri was defined as tumor in more than two cerebral lobes with or without involvement of the central parts of the cerebrum. The T2-weighted MRI (**a**) shows a glioma in the right frontal and temporal lob with extension into the left frontal lobe and affection of the left thalamus (*asterisk*). On the sagittal T2-weighted image (**b**) of another patient, gliomatosis is visible in enlarged frontal (*large arrow*) and parietal gyri along the corpus callosum. Via central cerebral structures the dorsal midbrain (*small arrow*) and tegmentum pontis are involved as well. On T1 after contrast (**c**) (same patient as in **a**), no enhancement is visible. No connection of T2-hypersignal is seen on (**d**) between the right temporal tumor and the T2-hyperintense signal predominantly in the right cerebellum (*arrow*). In a patient with a typical DIPG (**f**), a second glioma is seen on the T2-weighted image. It involves the left precentral gyrus (**e**)

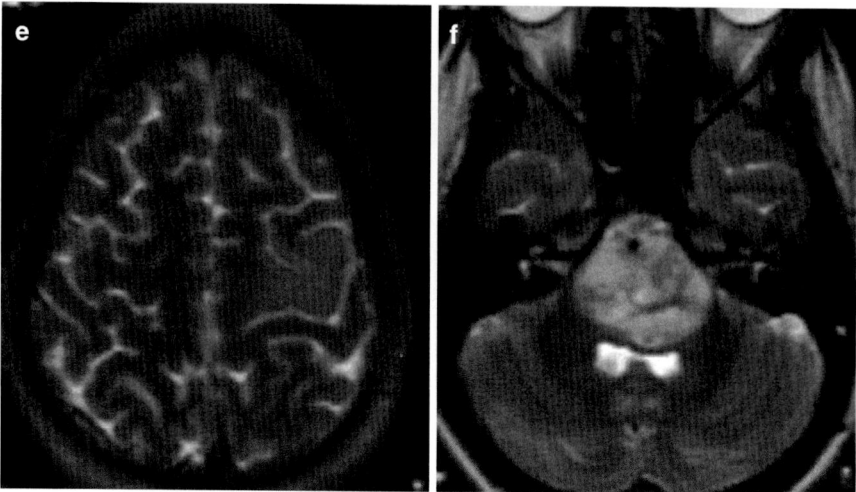

Fig. 3.15 (continued)

of the tectal plate itself but rather by the development of a triventricular hydrocephalus even in very small tumors due to their strategic localization close to the aqueduct. The patients are usually adapted to the hydrocephalus for many years. Consequently they are frequently diagnosed with a tectal glioma only by chance or by a decompensation of the increased CSF pressure equilibrium (Fig. 3.17). Therefore very young children or those with tectal plate symptoms are not found among children bearing typical tectal plate gliomas. In children with young age and local symptoms you should plan a rather short-term control (4–6 weeks) if histology is not clarified right away. We saw 2 PNETs in very young children mimicking tectal plate gliomas on imaging at the time of first MRI. However, extremely rapid growth and local symptoms like gaze abnormalities unmasked these tumors as highly malignant lesions later confirmed by histology. Of course all kinds of tumors can exceptionally be found in this area.

The typical tectal gliomas are usually smaller lesions with a high and mostly homogeneous T2-signal. Due to the usually massive ventricular dilatation, small tumors sometimes cannot be detected before a relief of hydrocephalus and tectal plate decompression was achieved. Contrast enhancement is more frequently missing. A relief of hydrocephalus by a third-ventriculostomy or a shunt is usually the only intervention needed for typical tectal gliomas. However, follow-up imaging is necessary to avoid a misleading imaging diagnosis and to identify the demand for treatment. Larger tumors, tumors extending into the thalamus, and those with contrast enhancement may need additional treatment like chemotherapy or irradiation after correction of increased CSF pressure [69].

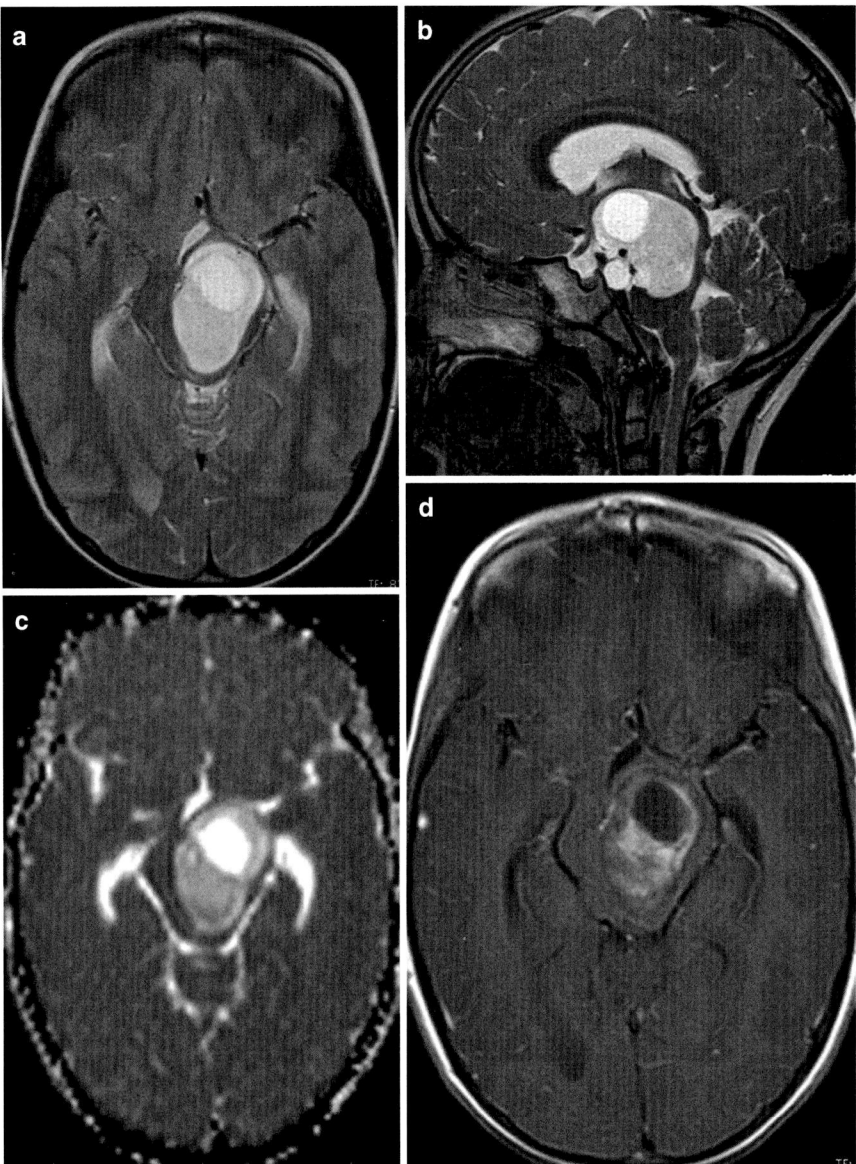

Fig. 3.16 A pilocytic astrocytoma in the left cerebral peduncle exhibits a sharp border on the axial T2-weighted MRI (**a**). On sagittal T2-weighted images (**b**) the main mass is confined to the preduncle only reaching the upper pons. Cellularity is low demonstrated by a high signal on ADC (**c**). The tumor enhances irregularly and intensively (**d**)

3.3.2.5   Diffuse Intrinsic Pontine Gliomas (DIPG)

Despite all treatment and scientific efforts DIPGs have remained the entity with the worst prognosis in children [70]. The median survival is below 1 year and the number of children surviving 3 years is very small. For this reason it is desirable to obtain tumor material to enhance further knowledge. This possibly may open new ways of treatment in the future [71]. For this reason the current strategy of only imaging diagnosis will probably be replaced in the future by regular biopsies although the histological diagnosis is usually well predictable by only MRI and clinical symptoms. The WHO grades of DIPG may vary from II to IV and cannot be differentiated by MRI. However, the course of disease, prognosis, and treatment does not depend on the individual WHO grades. For the imaging diagnosis of a DIPG, it is most important to define the main tumor site to be clearly centered in the pons (Fig. 3.18a, b). Diffuse high-grade gliomas can be found as well in the medulla

Fig. 3.17 The massive but not acute triventricular hydrocephalus in an older child is caused by a typical tectal glioma (no histological verification). The chronic hydrocephalus can be diagnosed due to a massive enlargement of the sella with vanished clinoid processes (*asterisk*)

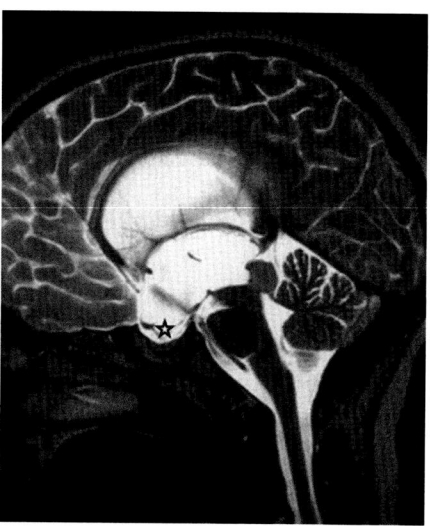

Fig. 3.18 (**a–j**) (**a**) on the sagittal T2-weighted MRI, a DIPG confirmed by biopsy resulting in a small defect with hemosiderin deposition in the edge is clearly centered in the pons. (**b**) On the sagittal T2-weighted MRI the histologically confirmed anaplastic ependymoma is growing from outside into the pons and is not an intrinsic lesion. A DIPG is covering more than half of the cross sectional area on this axial T2-weighted image (**c**). Sharp borders are rather frequently seen on T2-weighted MRI (**d**). The intrinsic growth of this glioma is demonstrated by a splitting of the pontine formatio reticularis on the coronal T2-weighted sequence (**e**). The suspicion of a pilocytic astrocytoma was raised by the dorsal cyst and confirmed by biopsy. The enhancement pattern on this postcontrast T1-sequence (**f**) is quite characteristic for a pilocytic astrocytoma. A focal pontine glioma in two different patients covers less than half of the cross-sectional area of the pons on T2-weighted images (**g, h**). Although the tumor is not enhancing (same patient as in **h**) on a post-contrast T1-weighted image (**i**), there seems to be a dorsal cyst. This feature is very much in favor of a pilocytic astrocytoma. In a child with NF-1 (**j**) as well high T2-signal areas in the cerebellum (NF-1 associated lesions) and an engulfment and signal increase in the pons is seen

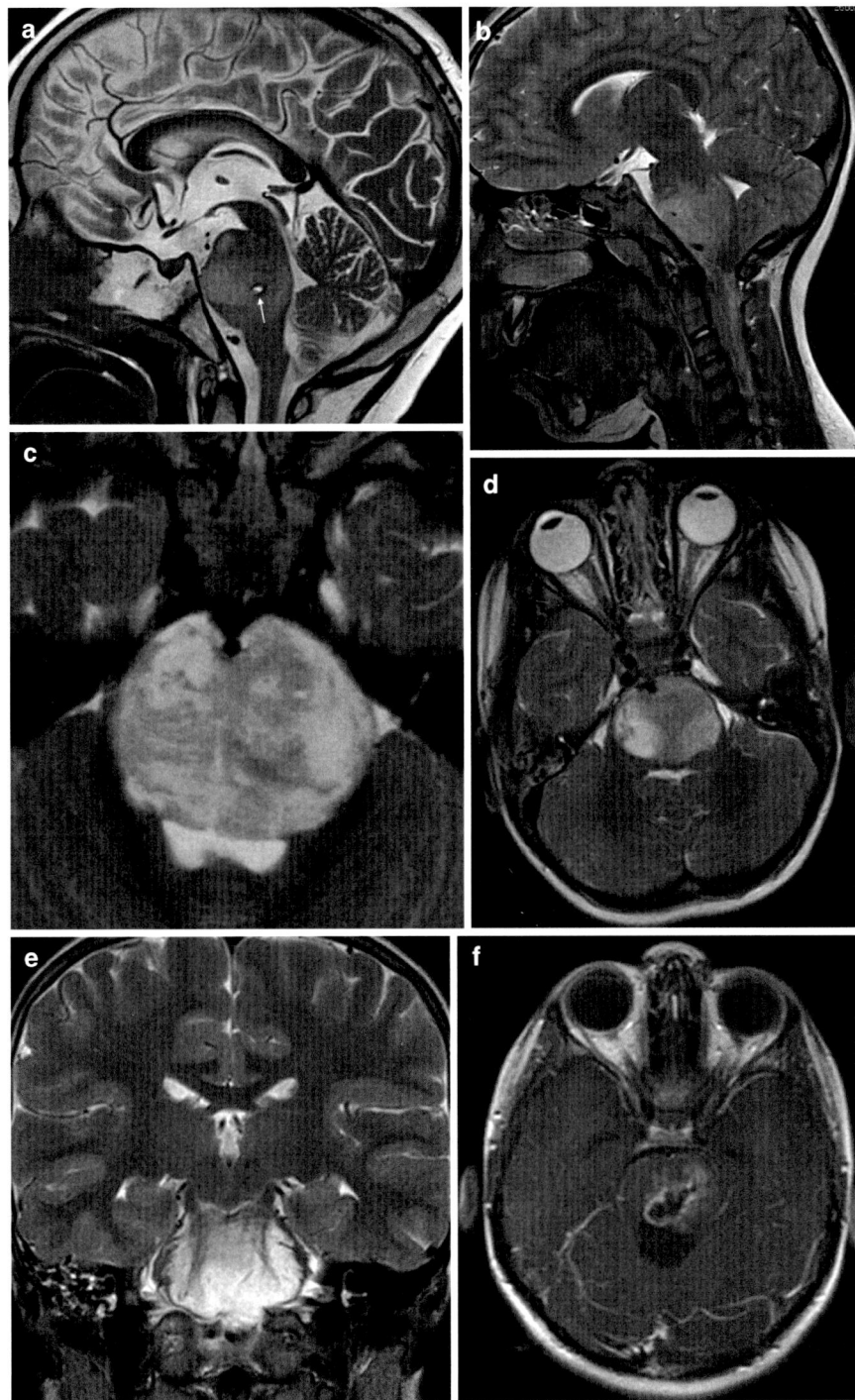

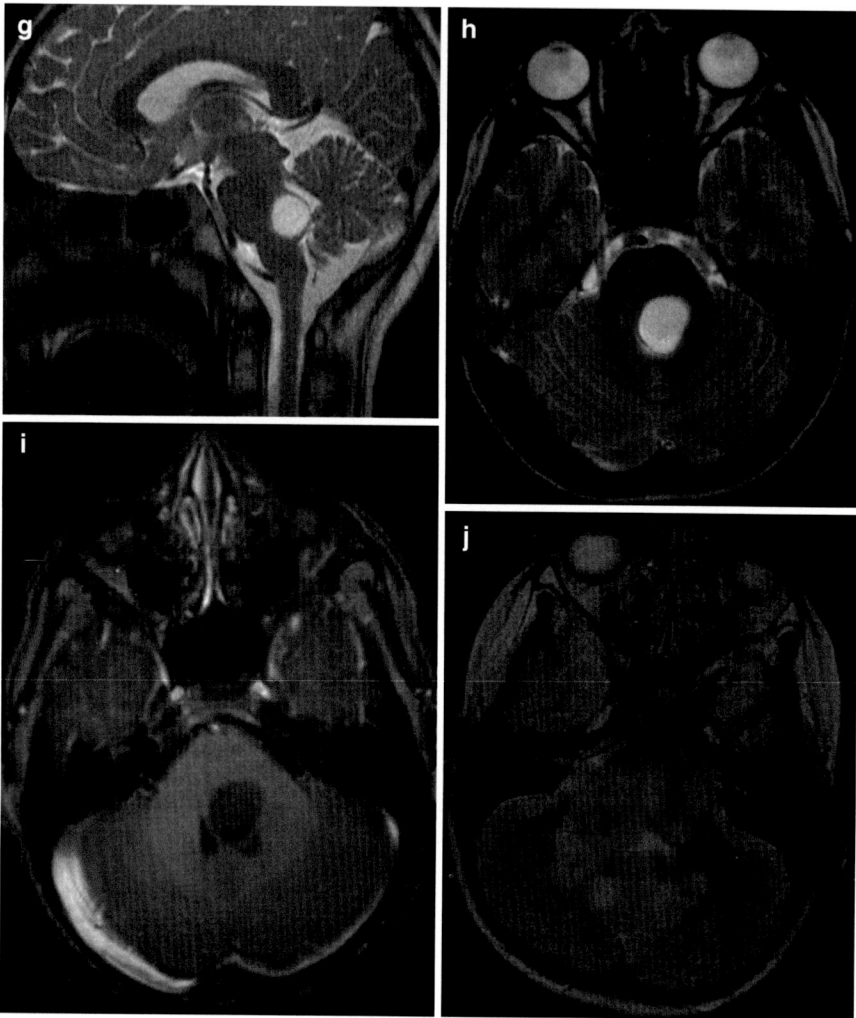

Fig. 3.18 (continued)

oblongata, but in these children a biopsy is indispensible to achieve a histological diagnosis with certainty. Usually a DIPG covers more that half of the pons [72] (Fig. 3.18c). Contrast behavior is variable. The borders may be very sharp on T2-weighted images (Fig. 3.18d). Usually as a sign of infiltrative growth the fibers of the formatio reticularis are seen as engulfed and split by the high T2-signal of the infiltrating tumor (Fig. 3.18e). Real cysts are not found and should warrant a histological clarification of the lesion because they are frequently found in pilocytic astrocytomas, which can grow in the pons as in all parts of the CNS (Fig. 3.18f). Also focal gliomas of the pons covering less than half of the cross sectional area should be closely watched or histologically clarified (Fig. 3.18h, i). Extension in inferior and more frequently superior direction or into the cerebellum is seen either at diagnosis or during follow-up. A perifocal edema cannot be distinguished from the tumor itself and the entire T2/FLAIR hyperintensity is considered tumor. Asymmetric growth is not unusual. If enhancement is present at the time of diagnosis it does not contradict the diagnosis of a DIPG. However, it has been described as a sign of a worse prognosis as well in our patient group as also in other larger treatment studies [73, 74]. Leptomeningeal dissemination is possible but rare compared to embryonal tumors at diagnosis and increases during follow-up [75]. As in all diffuse gliomas, further intracerebral tumors distant from the pons may be seen either synchronously or during follow-up [76] (Fig. 3.15e, f). During or soon after treatment the tumor may shrink and the high T2-signal may approximate to normal. A new reactive contrast enhancement within a DIPG is often found on the postradiation MRI and must not be interpreted as a sign of tumor progression during this phase of treatment.

In NF1, gliomas of the pons can imitate a DIPG on MRI (Fig. 3.18j). However, the clinical course in NF1 patients is much more favorable and a specific treatment is not initiated due to the fact that a tumor in the pons is present but rather depends on the course of disease and the patient's clinical complaints.

3.3.2.6 Gliomas of the Medulla Oblongata

While gliomas of the pons are not at all resectable, their dorsal exophytic counterpart in the medulla oblongata sometimes extending downwards into the spinal cord (Fig. 3.19a, b) is frequently considered to be decompressable by the experienced neurosurgeon. This is the initial method of choice for treating a dorsal exophytic, symptomatic glioma of the medulla oblongata and a good way to confirm the histology of a low-grade glioma [77, 78]. Most frequent histologies are pilocytic astrocytomas, gangliogliomas (Fig. 3.19c, d), and diffuse astrocytomas grade II in our patients. Contrast accumulation is variable.

3.4 Ependymomas

Ependymomas show different genetic alterations and behavior according to their localization [79]. In the posterior fossa they are the main differential diagnosis to MBs. They usually grow in close spatial relation to the ependymal lining in the posterior fossa either within the mainly lower parts of the ventricle or near the ependymal protrusions into the cerebellopontine angle (Fig. 3.20a, b). As they are tumors with a dense cellularity, the T2-signal is low in the solid parts of the tumor but usually not as low as in MB and free water diffusion may be impeded. The internal structure frequently shows rim enhancing cystic formations (necroses) with an elevated protein content. Inhomogeneity is predominant (Fig. 3.20a, b). Occasionally ependymomas are homogeneous on T2 or do not take up contrast [80] (Fig. 3.20c, d)

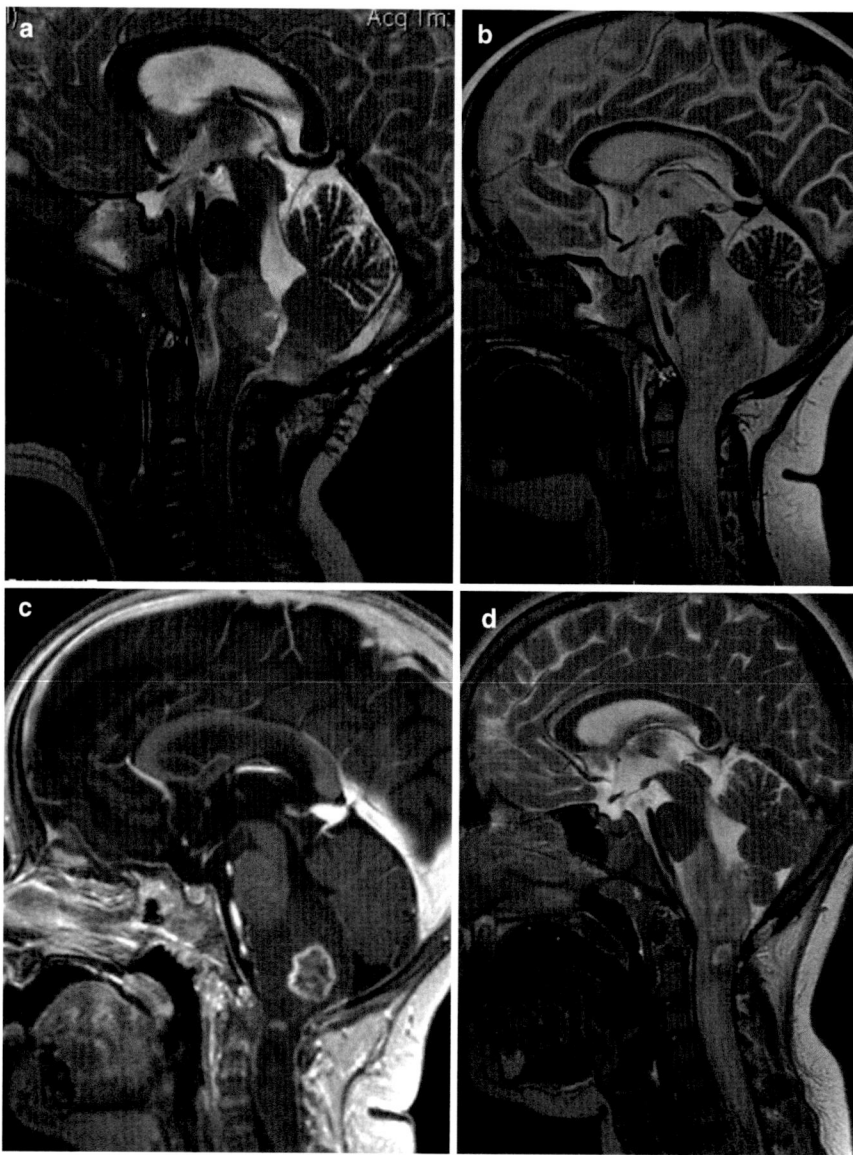

Fig. 3.19 In the medulla oblongata, diffuse tumors with a definite dorsal exophytic component are very frequently low-grade gliomas. They may involve only the medulla oblongata (as seen in **a**) or extend into the cervical cord (**b–e**) and are then called cervicomedullary tumors. Pilocytic astrocytomas (**b**, **c**) or diffuse astrocytomas WHO grade II are not well distinguishable from gangliogliomas (**d**, **e**). Contrast enhancement in gangliogliomas (**e**) is more frequently irregular and looking "infiltrative"

Fig. 3.19 (continued)

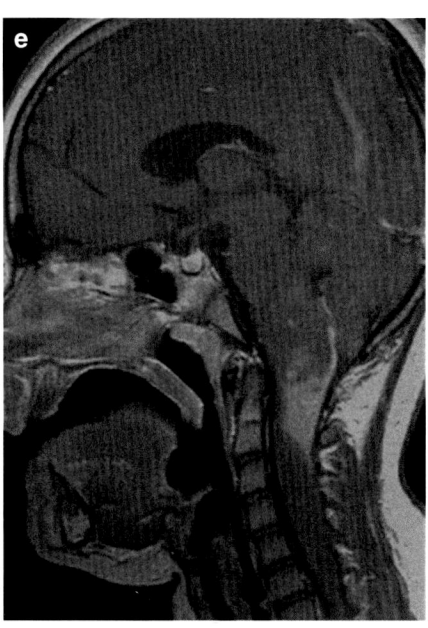

although enhancement is intense and striking in most ependymomas. The most characteristic feature is the so-called plastic growth pattern [81], which leads to an early sprouting out of the posterior fossa mainly into the spinal canal and the encasement of prepontine vessels and cranial nerve roots (Fig. 3.20e). Involvement of the foramen of Magendie is much more frequent (Fig. 3.20f) than in MB [80]. The encasing growth pattern is the main obstacle for a complete resection and a good outcome. Complete resection is an important precondition for cure in ependymomas.

In the supratentorial compartment, most ependymomas do not grow in the ventricles (Fig. 3.21a, b) but in the vicinity of the outer ventricular border within the brain parenchyma [82, 83]. Intraventricular growth is rarely found and was associated with lack of RELA fusion transcript genes in our patients. Especially supratentorially large cysts are frequent (Fig. 3.21c).

As well infra- as also supratentorial tumors rarely show leptomeningeal dissemination already at the time of diagnosis. During follow-up the incidence of dissemination in cranial ependymomas increases significantly and even isolated spinal deposits or isolated intraventricular nodules may be found (Fig. 3.21d). Therefore a complete screening of the CSF space may not be as important at diagnosis as it is during follow-up [84]. Nevertheless, the standard staging examination in ependymomas includes a complete spinal MRI. Spinal ependymomas in children are mainly myxopapillary WHO grade I tumors of the filum terminale. They behave differently than the WHO grade II and III tumors affecting the brain. However,

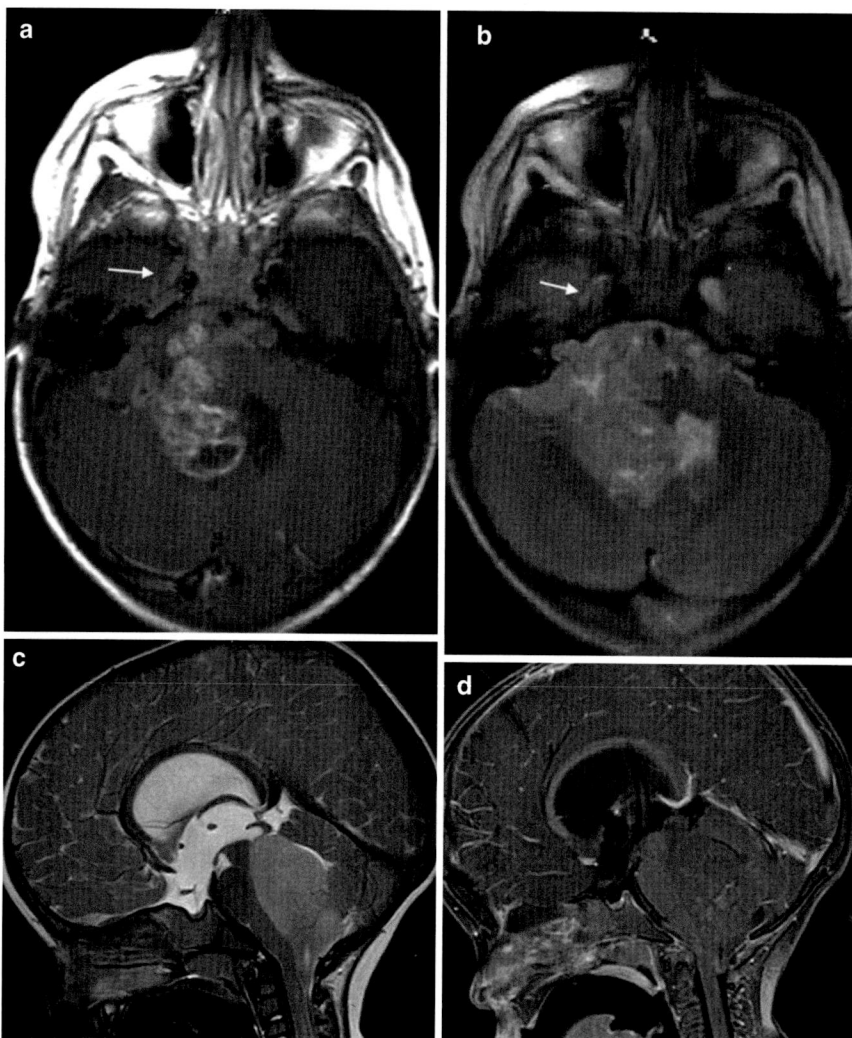

Fig. 3.20 Ependymomas in the posterior fossa frequently show irregular but rather intense contrast enhancement and an inhomogeneous internal structure with cyst-like components like this tumor arising from the right cerebellopontine angle on axial T1-weighted postcontrast (**a**) and T2-weighted (**b**) images. The "plastic" growth pattern led to a surrounding of the pontine structures and an infiltration into the internal auditory canal and even Meckels' cave on the right hand side (*arrow*). Also homogeneous tumors without significant enhancement (**c, d**) may be seen. An early extension into the spinal canal is frequent (**e**) and the foramen of Magendie is frequently involved as seen on a sagittal CISS image (**f**)

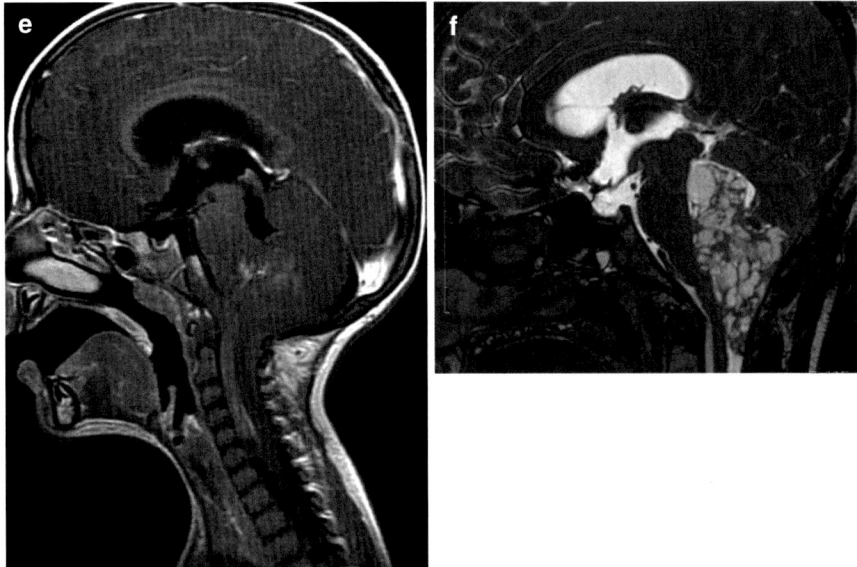

Fig. 3.20 (continued)

myxopapillary ependymomas tend to develop not only recurrences but also metastases (Fig. 3.21e, f) and a complete imaging of the CSF space in defined intervals is recommended [85, 86].

3.5 Germ Cell Tumors

Germinomas are the most frequent germ cell tumors. The predominant localization is the pineal region. Second most frequently they are found in the suprasellar area [87]. The typical age at diagnosis is in the second and third decade and males predominate. Germ cell tumors and germinomas have a high cell density and nucleus/plasma-relation and are therefore similar to gray matter on T2 [61] with a restricted diffusion [88] (Fig. 3.22a, b). More than 95 % of our tumors showed mostly intense contrast enhancement (Fig. 3.22c). Intense enhancement is also seen in their metastases in the CSF or along the subependymal lining of the ventricles (Fig. 3.22d). A quite distinct picture is found if germinomas grow in the basal ganglia. The clinical picture is dominated by a slowly progressing hemiparesis. The affected side of the basal ganglia rather shows atrophic changes than a mass lesion combined with a highly cellular lesion as derivable from hyperdense CT-density values and iso- or hypointense T2-signals sometimes showing contrast uptake [89] (Fig. 3.22e–h). The prognosis for a reduction of symptoms after treatment is worse in this group. Bifocal tumor growth meaning synchronous tumors in the pineal and suprasellar area is not infrequent (10–25 % in our database) and not considered as disseminated [90] (Fig. 3.22c). Outside the pineal, suprasellar, and basal ganglia region, they rarely originate from any part of the brain and spinal cord and are then indistinguishable from other brain tumors. We saw one germinoma in the diencephalon, one in the brain stem and two in the spinal cord in about 230 patients. Histology can only be clarified by biopsy or resection in these unusual cases. Germinomas are usually quite homogeneous tumors and are

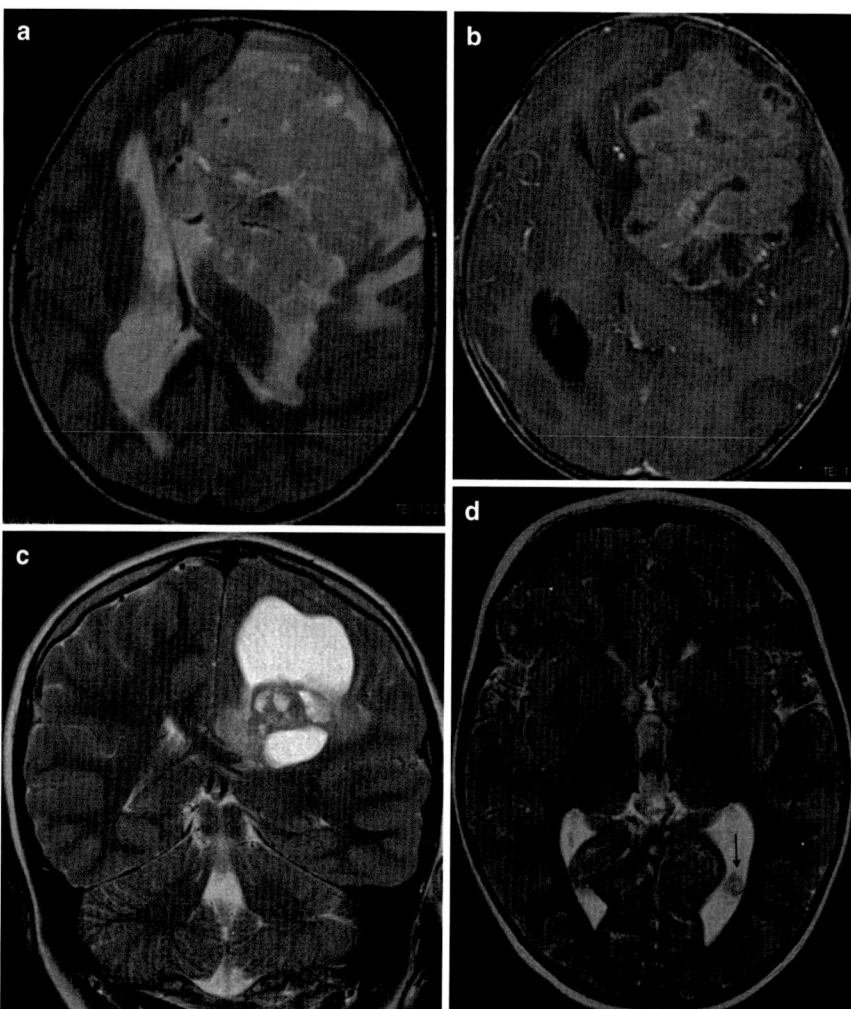

Fig. 3.21 Supratentorial ependymomas are tumors with a high cell density with an intermediate to low T2-signal and usually growing outside in ventricles (**a, b**). Larger cysts (different child in (**c**) then in (**a, b**)) are not rare (**c**). During follow-up a CSF-dissemination in a different patient may occur as seen by a inhomogeneous nodule in the left lateral ventricle (*arrow* on **d**). A myxopapillary ependymoma of the filum terminale (**e**) was completely resected. After some time small disseminated nodules (*arrows*) recurred without a local recurrence of the tumor (**f**)

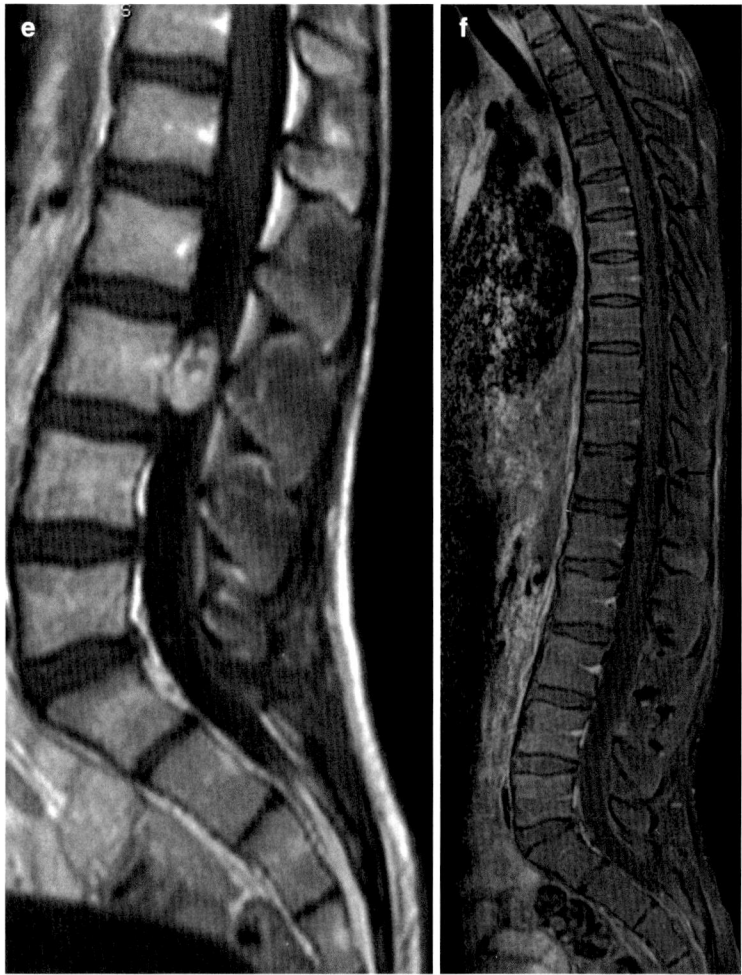

Fig. 3.21 (continued)

nonsecreting tumors. Secreting germ cell tumors are defined by a diagnosis of increased levels of human chorion gonadotropin (hCG) and alpha1-fetoprotein (AFP) in the serum and/or CSF. Secreting tumors are usually composed of several histological varieties frequently also including germinoma parts. They bear a more unfavorable prognosis and treatment differs from pure germinomas [91]. Therefore in case of a suspected germ cell tumor, the examination of CSF and blood serum plays a very important role and only after this clarification biopsy or surgery should be considered. In secreting germ cell tumors treatment may be started after a completed staging for CSF dissemination without a histological clarification. In nonsecreting tumors, only bifocal tumors are considered as germinomas and may also be treated without histology. In all other tumors, a histological clarification preferably by biopsy is necessary. Biopsy is preferred to attempted complete resection in these frequently well treatment

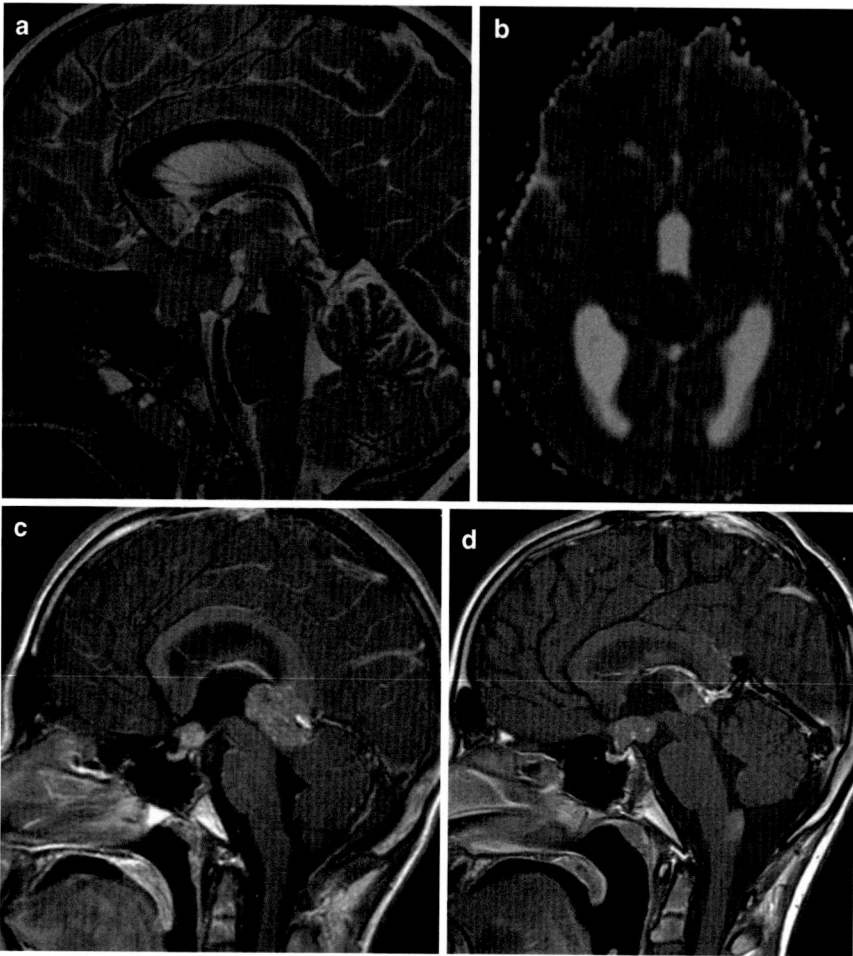

Fig. 3.22 MRIs from different patients: The T2-signal of a bifocal germ cell tumor (**a**) is comparable to gray matter. High cell density leads to a dark ADC (**b**) of a tumor in the pineal region. A bifocal localization in the suprasellar and pineal region (**a** and **c**) is not considered as a disseminated tumor and nearly all germ cell tumors enhance (**c**). Metastases also enhance (in **d** at the level of the obex). A basal ganglia germ cell tumor (**e–h**) can be suspected if atrophic changes in the basal ganglia are combined with hyperdense CT values (**h**), a dark ADC (**g**) of the tumor and some contrast enhancement (**f**). Irregular and inhomogeneous T2- (**i**) and T1-signals (**j**) are more frequent in nongerminomatous germ cell tumors as shown in this secreting tumor. A frequent route of dissemination in germ cell tumors is along the borders here shown in the lateral ventricles (**k**) or even the optic nerve sheaths (**l**) in another child. These extensions even if in continuity with the primary tumor are considered as dissemination in the SIOP-CNS-GCT study. Response assessment in this study is sometime not possible without doubt because the affected areas like the pituitary stalk and the pineal gland (*arrow*) may vary in normal size between individuals. We advice a short term control to prove additional shrinkage and therefore rendering the first examination as very good partial response (**n**) but not complete response (**o**). (**m**, MRI before treatment (**n**), after the first part of treatment (**o**), after further 4 weeks of treatment). Loss of pituitary bright spot on nonenhanced T1-weighted sagittal slices (SL 2–3 mm) in two different patients (**p**, **q**) with "unexplained" diabetes insipidus and thickened pituitary stalk. Both patients showed growth of a suprasellar germ cell tumor on follow-up. Brighter structure after contrast enhancement (**r**, **s**) anterior to an intra- and suprasellar germinoma in two different patients probably representing the anterior pituitary (*arrow*)

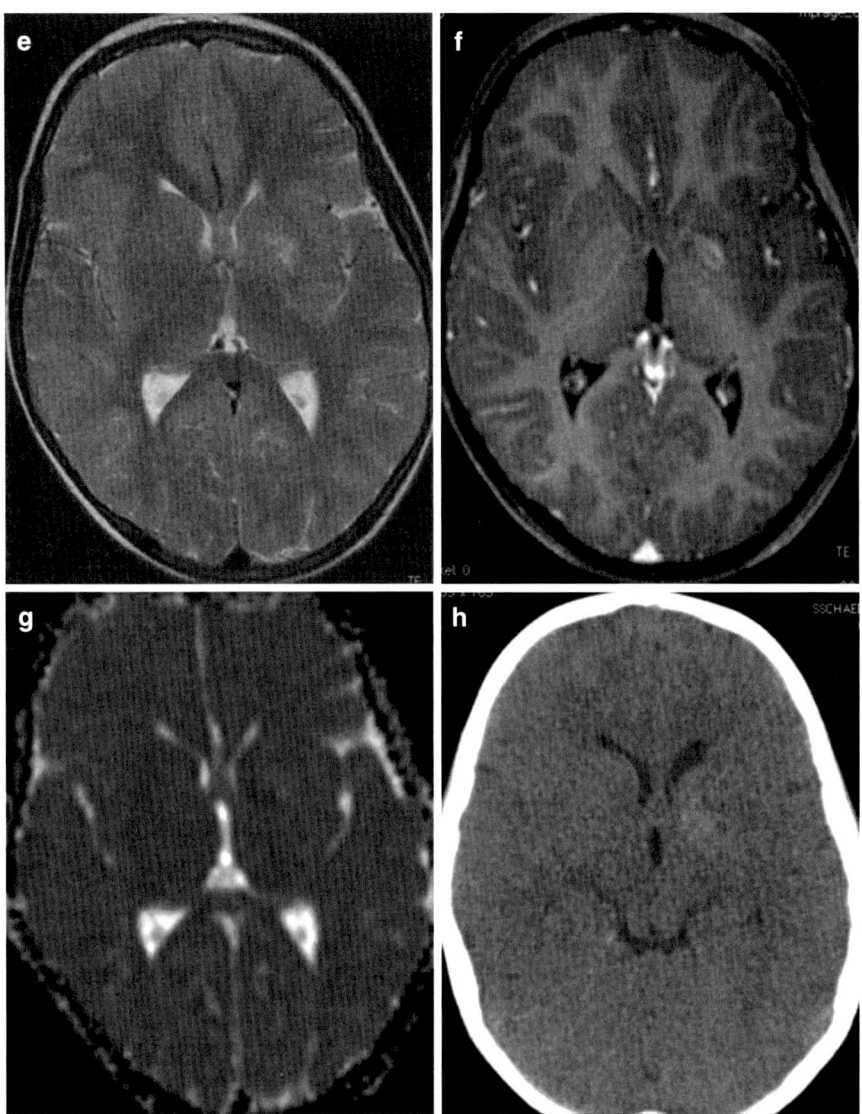

Fig. 3.22 (continued)

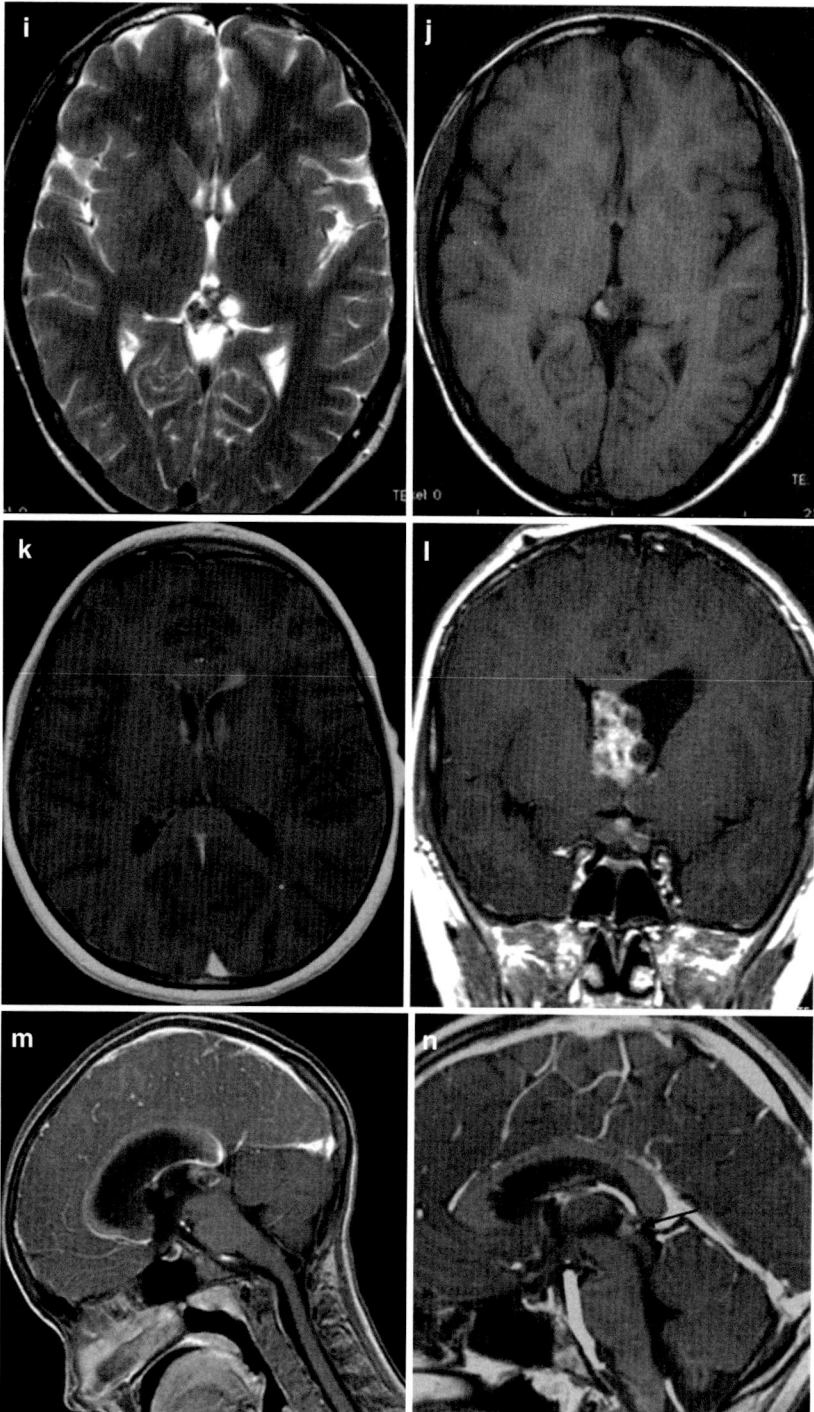

Fig. 3.22 (continued)

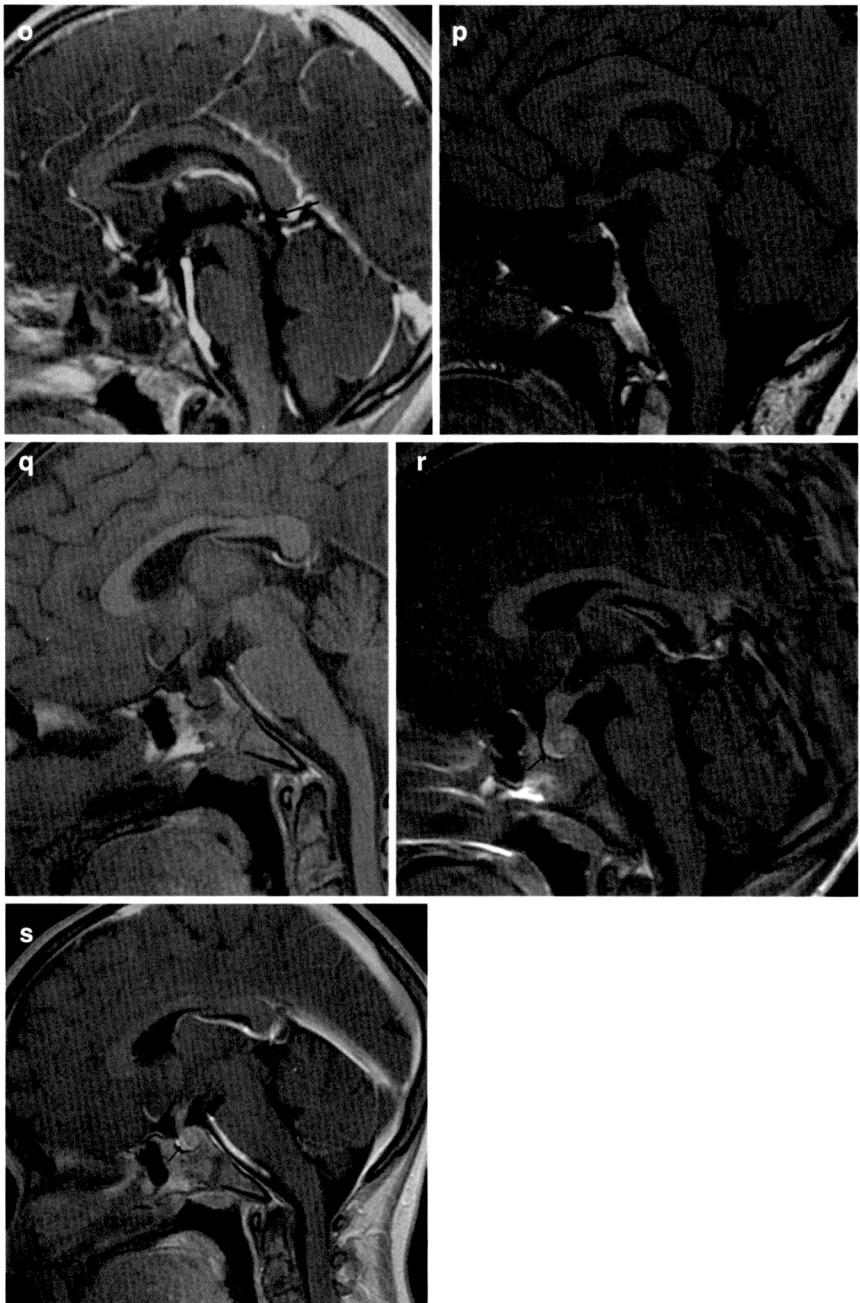

Fig. 3.22 (continued)

responsive tumors in a delicate localization. Secreting and mixed germ cell tumors usually contain teratoma parts, which are inhomogeneous tumors containing larger cysts (Fig. 3.22i, j). After treatment usually the teratoma part persists without further change and has to be resected to achieve complete response. However, surgery is usually easier after a significant reduction of size [92].

A frequent and characteristic way of dissemination is an extension along the ventricular borders subependymally or along the optic nerve sheaths [93] (Fig. 3.22k, l). Germ cell tumors with a similar extension are considered as disseminated in the ongoing SIOP CNS-GCT study even if there is a direct contact to the primary tumor.

As germ cell tumors affect structures that physiologically enhance, like the pituitary stalk and the pineal gland which do not have a clear cutoff to a normal size in an individual patient, it is sometimes hard or even impossible to separate a very good partial response with a nearly complete regression of the tumor from a true complete response. We solve this problem for the ongoing SIOP-CNS-GCT study with a follow-up examination. If there is a further reduction during treatment we then retrospectively can diagnose a very good partial response. But if the lesion remains in the same size we can conclude that this was a true complete response already at the time of the previous MRI (Fig. 3.22m–o). Contrast enhancement is reliable and if enhancement is completely gone we diagnose a complete remission even if T2-signal abnormalities persist and are then considered scar tissue.

Germ cell tumors of the suprasellar region may be slowly growing and frequently cause a disturbance of the posterior pituitary lobe resulting in the clinical picture of a diabetes insipidus [94–96]. As the size of the pituitary stalk cannot be predicted in an individual patient, sometimes a slowly growing borderline or slightly thickened stalk is seen on MRI [97]. An indication of tumor growth in the pituitary stalk is the loss of the normal bright signal of the posterior pituitary lobe on unenhanced T1-weighted images [98] (Fig. 3.22p, q). We have the impression that small germ cell tumors arise from the posterior pituitary lobe and grow from there upward to the floor of the third ventricle. The displaced and compressed anterior pituitary lobe can be visualized in front of the tumor in early cases (Fig. 3.22r, s). In our database we did not find the posterior bright spot in nearly all germ cell tumors in suprasellar localization. Unfortunately, this diagnostic tool can only be used if imaging is performed according to our guideline of an ideal imaging in suprasellar lesions including sagittal thin slice T1-sequences before the injection of contrast medium. We prefer SE or TSE in 2–3 mm thickness to MPR sequences even if thinner slice lengths are possible. (See Sect. 3.2.)

3.6   Craniopharyngiomas

In the suprasellar region, craniopharyngiomas are the most frequent nonglial tumors in children. Boys and girls are equally affected and the peak incidence is in the first decade. Craniopharyngiomas are rare tumors representing only 1.2–4.6 % [99] of intracranial tumors at all. They are divided into two histological subtypes with different origin, development, and morphology: the adamantinous and the papillary subtype. The later is presumably induced by metaplastic changes of buccal mucosa premordia in the Rathke cleft and pouch and affects only adults with a peak incidence in the fifth and sixth decade. Adamantinous craniopharyngiomas are found in all ages but are the only craniopharyngiomas in children and adolescents. Their origin is cell remnants of teeth premordia in the Rathke pouch and duct, a tubular later in development involuted structure. Through Rathke's duct, the anterior pituitary forms meeting the posterior pituitary an evagination from the floor of the third ventricle to form the united pituitary gland [100]. The typical localization of craniopharyngiomas is the intra- and suprasellar region. Less frequently they arise only in the suprasellar position and even rarer exclusively intrasellarly (intrasellar 4 %, suprasellar 25 %, and intra-/suprasellar 71 % in our database). Exceptionally rare and unexplained are anecdotal reports of craniopharyngiomas arising in other localizations as, e.g., the fourth ventricle. Craniopharyngiomas are malformative tumors and do not disseminate. Rare reports on second tumors after resection mainly in the surgical access are thought to arise from implantation of tumor during surgery [101]. This can also explain drop "metastases" in the spinal canal. Adamantinous craniopharyngiomas are predominantly cystic tumors. Macroscopically the cysts frequently contain a fluid resembling machine-oil called colloid. On MRI colloid is characterized by a hyperintense signal on T1-weighted images before contrast enhancement and is quite characteristic (Fig. 3.23a). Cyst walls usually enhance and the histological hallmark of adamantinous craniopharyngiomas so-called wet keratin eventually calcifies resulting to a high proportion of calcifications (91 % in our database; Fig. 3.23b). A so-called 90 %-rule defines 90 % of cysts, calcifications, and cyst wall enhancement in adamantinous craniopharyngiomas [102] (Fig. 3.23c). On the contrary papillary tumors, which do not occur during childhood, do not calcify and are predominantly solid [59].

As in the other suprasellar tumors the bright pituitary spot is of differential diagnostic value. However, it depends on the individual localization and the size of the tumor if the bright posterior spot on unenhanced T1-weighted images can be seen (Fig. 3.23d, e). Usually the size of the pituitary is abnormally atrophic corresponding to a smaller size of children compared to normal controls already several years before the diagnosis of the tumor [103].

Rarely other lesions affect the pituitary and the stalk. Inflammations like hypophysitis are rare and cannot be diagnosed without histology. Langerhans cell histiocytosis (LCH) can affect the pituitary stalk and is an unclear disease (Fig. 3.24a). In case of a suspicion, a whole body MRI should be initiated to rule out the most frequently coexisting bone lesions. If they are not found, LCH is not a probable diagnosis. Hypothalamic hamartomas are rare malformations resembling abnormal brain with signal intensities comparable to gray matter (Fig. 3.24b).

The differential diagnoses to craniopharyngiomas besides true tumors like chiasmal LGGs and germ cell tumors are Rathke-cleft cysts and xanthogranulomas. Rathke cleft cysts can imitate small craniopharyngiomas perfectly and are cystic lesions in an intra-/suprasellar position (Fig. 3.24c). Xanthogranulomas are not considered tumors [104] and therefore not included in the WHO classi-

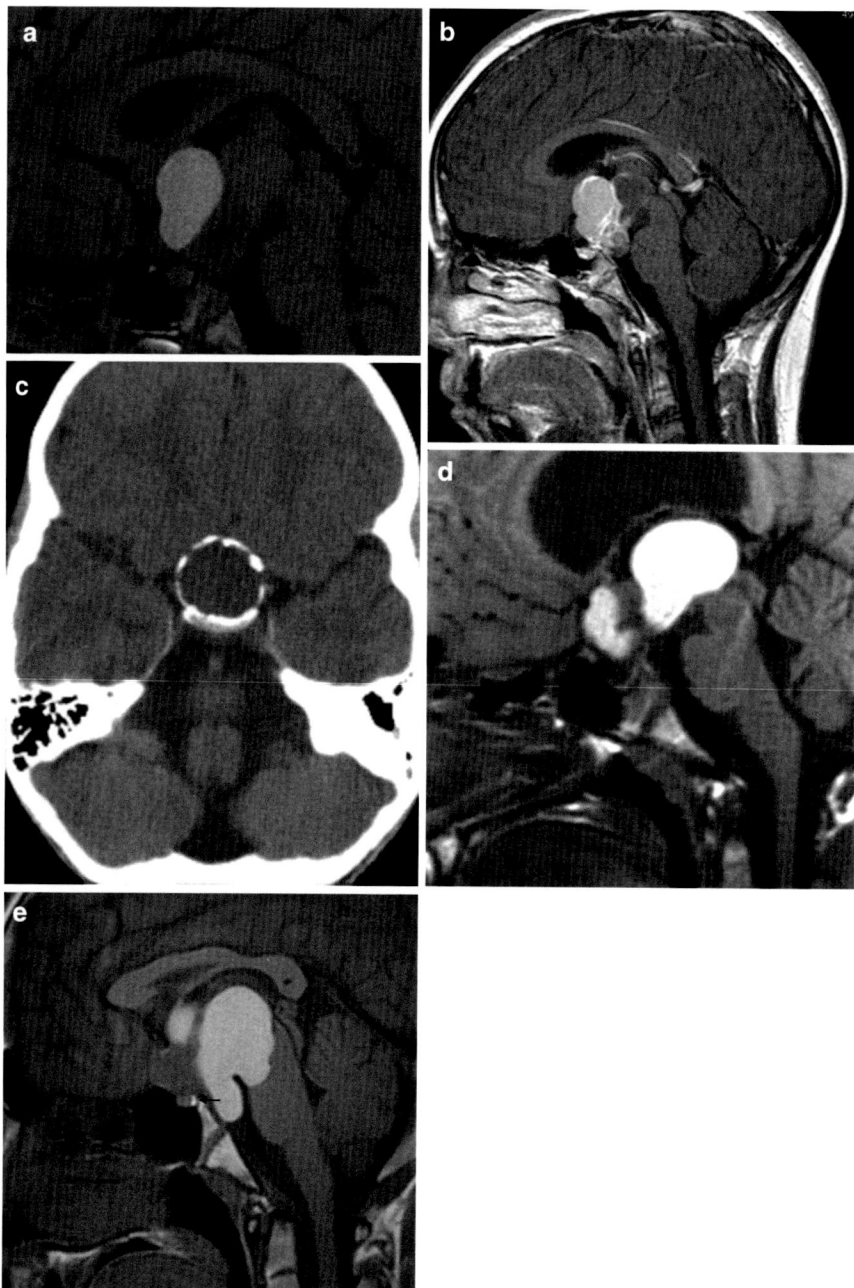

Fig. 3.23 Colloid is the content of one of the multiple cysts in a large craniopharyngioma (**a**). The walls of cysts show enhancement (**b**). Thick ring-like calcification on CT (**c**) in the cyst walls. Coarse calcifications are characteristic of adamantinous craniopharyngiomas. The loss of the bright posterior pituitary spot in a very atrophic pituitary gland is caused by a suprasellar cranio-pharyngioma (**d**). In another patient despite a large suprasellar craniopharyngioma the bright spot on unenhanced T1-weighted MRI (*arrow*) is preserved (**e**)

fication. They can be found in other parts of the brain, skull base, and body and are characterized by residues of bleeding leading to a primarily high signal on T1-weighted images in all our cases (Fig. 3.24d). However, a differentiation from colloid is not possible and small craniopharyngiomas cannot be distin-

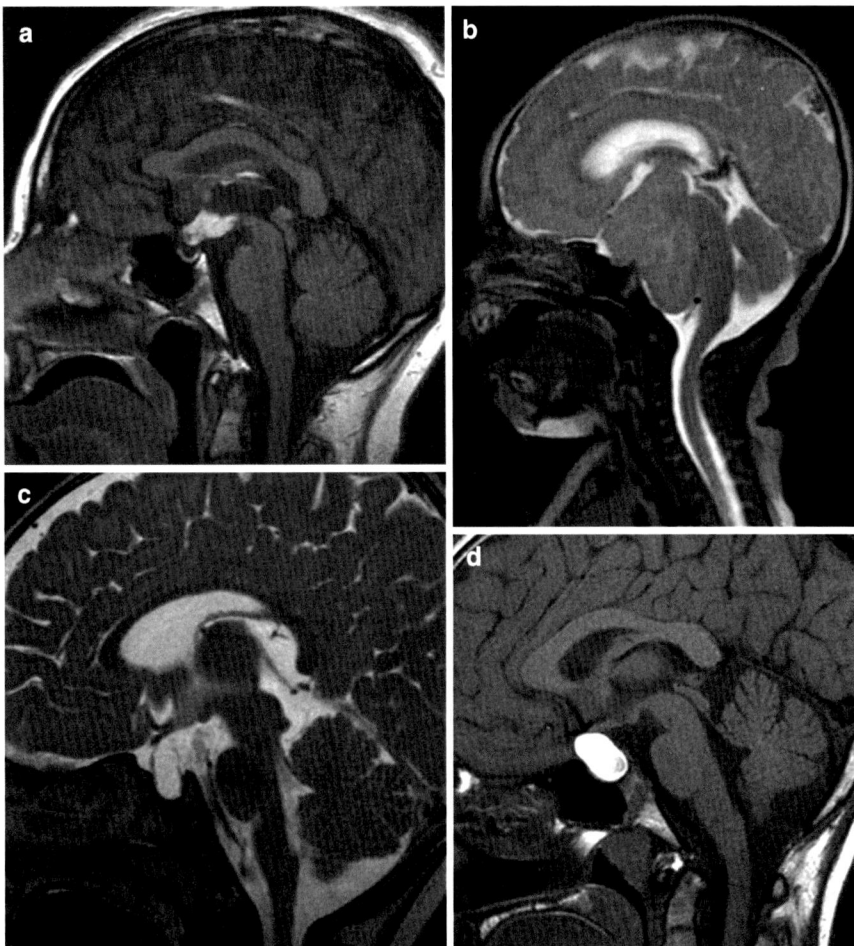

Fig. 3.24 A Langerhans cell histiocytosis in the suprasellar area cannot be differentiated from a germ cell tumor (**a**). Note also the pituitary atrophy. Search for additional bone and organ lesions. In a hypothalamic hamartoma, a mass with irregular gyrus-like pattern mimics abnormal brain (**b**). Rathke cysts (**c**) are intra- and suprasellar cystic lesions that cannot be differentiated from small purely cystic craniopharyngiomas. In xanthogranulomas (**d**) of the intra- and suprasellar region the high signal on unenhanced T1-weighted MRI is characteristic. On pathology this is explained by blood degradation products (met-hemoglobin). Development of a recurrence around a tiny residual calcification, visible on a plain CT (**e**) but not seen on the postoperative MRI (**f**) after resection of an adamantinous craniopharyngioma. The cystic recurrence (**g**) evolved exactly in the position of the residual calcification several months after surgery

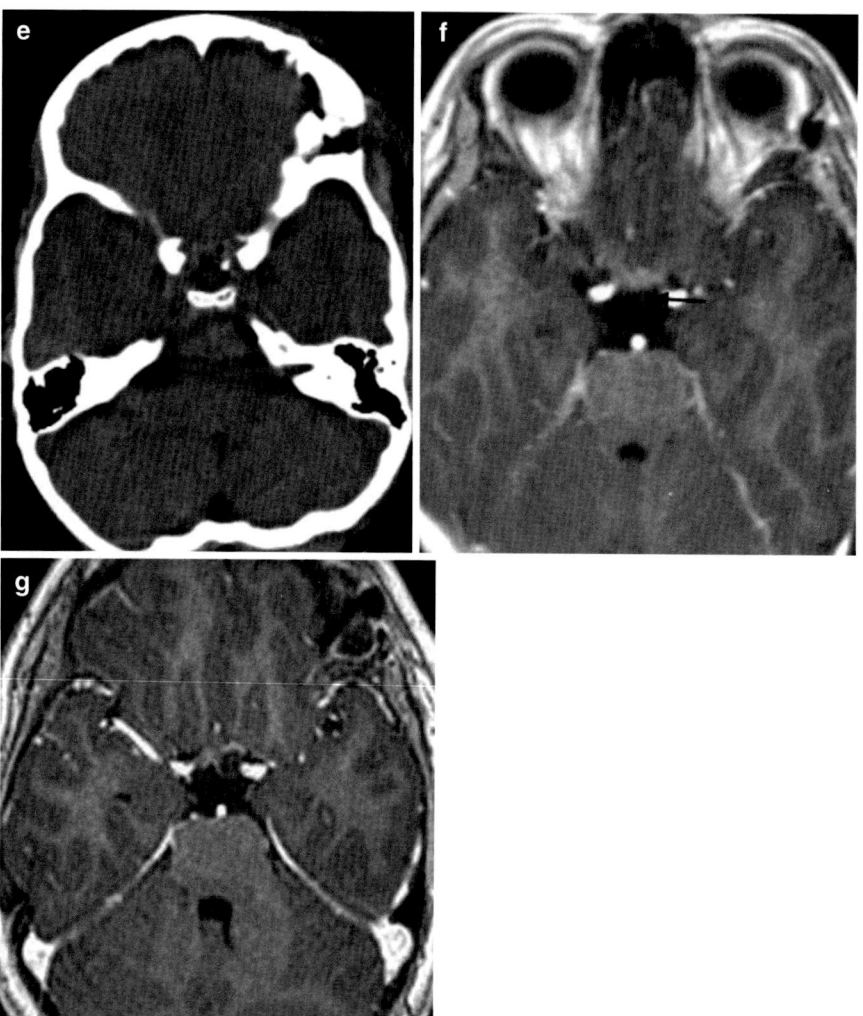

Fig. 3.24 (continued)

guished. In a report from Japan [105], a lack of calcification in five xantho-granulomas was thought to be a possibility for a differentiation from craniopharyngiomas. However, in our eight CTs of xanthogranulomas, we found five without and three containing calcifications. Thus the lack or existence of calcifications does not seem to help.

The regular early postoperative MRI (performed within 24–48 h after surgery, see also the chapter postoperative MRI) is frequently rather unclear, because craniopharyngiomas like pituitary adenomas or meningeomas are extraaxial tumors and the dura in and surrounding the surgical region shows immediate enhancement and may lead to the false impression of a residual tumor. We postpone the decision on a residual tumor in unclear MRI images to 2–3 months after surgery. Even if the postoperative MRI does not show a suspicion of a residual tumor, a residual calcification may remain undetected by MRI. The guidelines for imaging in the ongoing craniopharyngioma study contain the advice to perform a postoperative, unenhanced CT only of the tumor region avoiding to touch the eye lenses. With the means of this CT in a tumor free postoperative MRI a persisting calcification should be picked up under the assumption that a residual calcification signifies a residual tumor. Ellioth and coworkers [106] discussed this problem and reported that small residual calcifications (<2 mm) do not lead to an increased rate of relapses compared to postoperative sites without residual calcifications. We cannot contradict because in our database postoperative CTs are only scarce despite the fact that the postoperative MRI did not show a residual tumor. Contrary to the study guidelines, CTs are not performed fearing the inherent radiation in pediatric patients. However, we saw one patient with a tiny calcification, which was not detectable on his tumor-free postoperative MRI. In this patient, after some months a relapse occurred exactly around the tiny calcification (Fig. 3.24e–g).

Craniopharyngiomas tend to compromise the hypothalamus. Damage to this brain area either by the tumor itself or the surgical resection frequently leads to severe impairment of the quality of life by development of massive obesity. Adipositas together with hormonal deficiencies leads to severe metabolic syndromes and early deaths mostly from cardiovascular complications. It was recognized that patients with a compromise of the posterior hypothalamic nuclei are in danger of more severe side effects than those with a compression or damage of the anterior hypothalamus [107]. The surgical attitude to achieve a complete resection (whenever possible) is now changing to a staged resection or cysts treatment without touching the posterior hypothalamus (whenever possible) to avoid these devastating consequences [108] (Fig. 3.25a, b). Several classifications exist to identify the high-risk group [109, 110]. In the German craniopharyngioma-studies we use the level of the mammillary bodies to separate the anterior from the posterior hypothalamus (Fig. 3.25c). The increase in the body mass index (BMI) correlates well to the thickness of the nuchal fat fold that can be measured on T1-weighted images on MRI (personal communication Prof. H. Müller Oldenburg, Germany, leader of the German craniopharyngioma study). Unfortunately, we also see increasingly frequently such a rapidly developing subcutaneous fat depositions in children after partial resections of chiasmatic gliomas or germ cell tumors (Fig. 3.25d, e). The rapid development of adipositas in operated chiasmal glioma or germ cell tumor patients is probably also due to a damage of the hypothalamic nuclei in analogy to craniopharyngiomas.

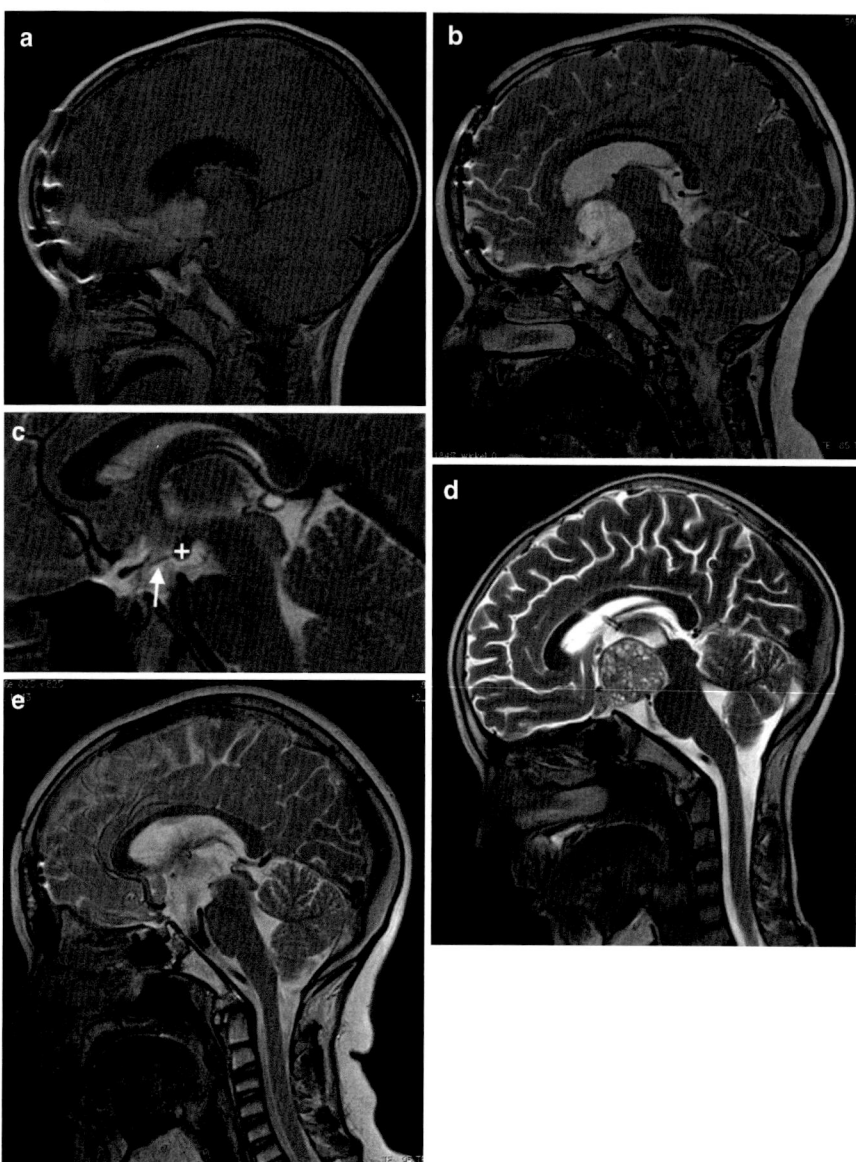

Fig. 3.25 Development of hypothalamic obesity demonstrated by the thickness of the subcutaneous fat in the dorsal neck in a patient after subfrontal resection of a craniopharyngioma. The early postoperative MRI (**a**) shows surgical changes in the access route in a slim girl. After only 3 months the thickness of the subcutaneous fat has at least doubled (**b**). Note the large defect after extensive resection. Anatomic illustration of the anterior hypothalamus (in front of the mammillary bodies) and the posterior hypothalamus (including the mammillary bodies and behind) in a patient with a small tectal glioma (**c**). The floor of the third ventricle is clearly seen as a thin line (*arrow*) and the normal mammillary bodies are marked with a white cross. Note also a small, triangular intermediate lobe cyst in the pituitary. This must not be diagnosed as a pathologic structure but as a harmless incidental finding. Hypothalamic obesity is not exclusive for craniopharyngiomas but rather a general consequence of damage to the hypothalamus. After complete resection (**d**: preoperative MRI) of a secreting germ cell tumor the subcutaneous fat has considerably increased after only 8 months (**e**). Note the large defect in the floor of the third ventricle and the tiny mammillary bodies behind the defect

◀───

3.7 Choroid Plexus Tumors

Choroid plexus tumors are rare overall (0.3–0.6 % of all brain tumors) but represent 2–4 % of tumors in children and 10–20 % of tumors in the first year of life [111]. Three grades of malignancy are found with plexus papillomas representing WHO grade I (Fig. 3.26a–f), atypical plexus papillomas WHO grade II (Fig. 3.26g, h), and choroid plexus carcinomas WHO grade III (Fig. 3.26i, j). Papillomas are about 5 times more frequent than carcinomas. A correct differentiation between the three possible entities is not always possible although the typical papilloma is a circumscribed, sharply delimited, cauliflower-like tumor attached to the ventricular plexus with intense contrast enhancement. A ventricular dilatation at diagnosis may be due to hyperproduction of CSF or a blockage of the CSF pathways. Infiltration of the ventricular wall or the brain parenchyma is unusual. Carcinomas are typically larger and inhomogeneous tumors, which infiltrate into the brain and lead to a perifocal edema. Leptomeningeal metastases do not exclude the diagnosis of a papilloma, although carcinomas disseminate more frequently (Fig. 3.26k, l). Not infrequent in plexus carcinomas is a contrast enhancement pattern resembling AT/RTs. Interestingly also on neuropathology AT/RTs are a possible differential diagnosis to plexus carcinomas [112, 113].

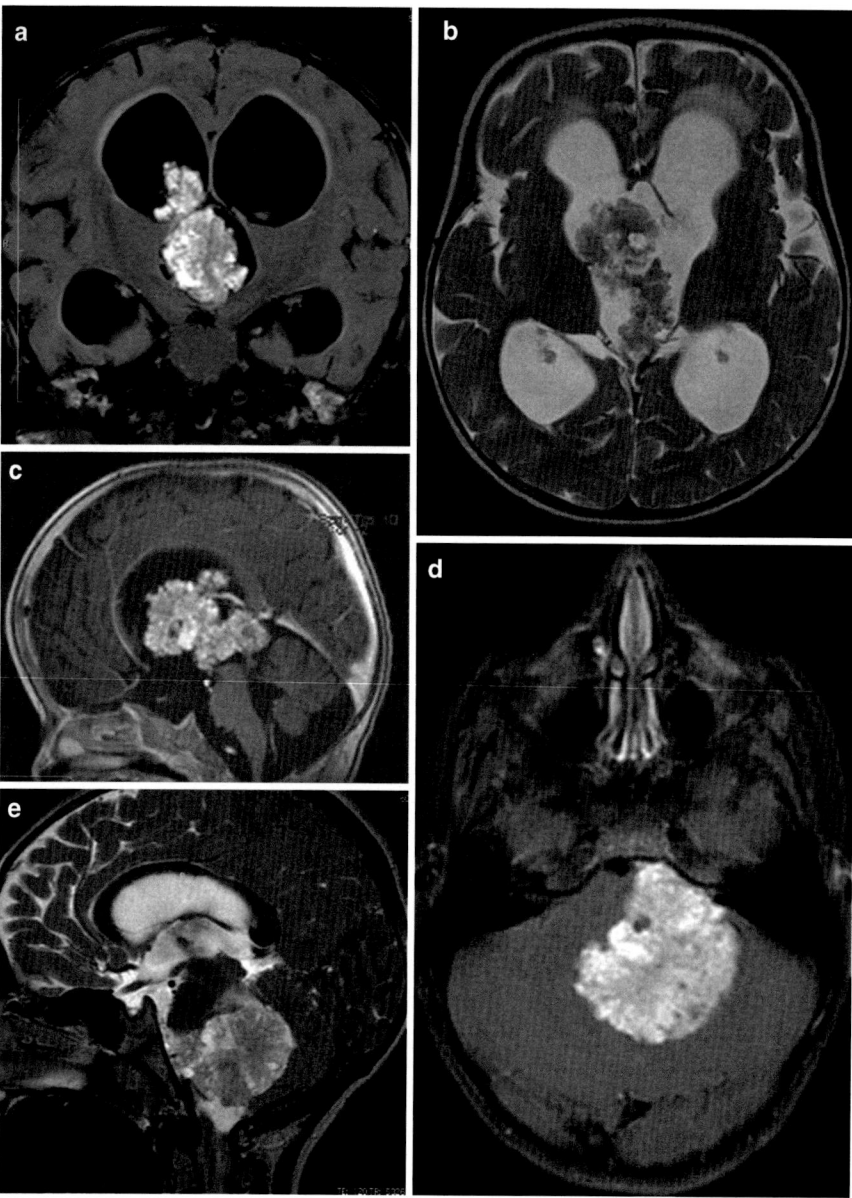

Fig. 3.26 (a–m) A papilloma of the plexus in the third ventricle in a young child shows the typical cauliflower aspect and a hydrocephalus (**a–c**). In an adolescent (**d–f**) a papilloma in the fourth ventricle is localized in the left cerebellopontine angle and could be mistaken for a WNT-MB due to its location. However, there is no restricted diffusion (**f**) with a bright ADC rendering a highly cellular tumor like an MB unlikely. The atypical PPL in a young child (**g, h**) cannot be distinguished from the typical case on (**a–c**). In a plexus carcinoma (**i–k**) there is obvious infiltration of the temporal lobe with edema, an indistinct border and an irregular structure. Note also the nodular leptomeningeal metastasis in the fourth ventricle (**j**). There were also other metastases not shown on the pictures. In a young adult with a typical, completely resected PPL (**l**) spinal leptomeningeal metastases (**m**) persist completely unchanged on follow-up for several years despite treatment with chemotherapy some years ago

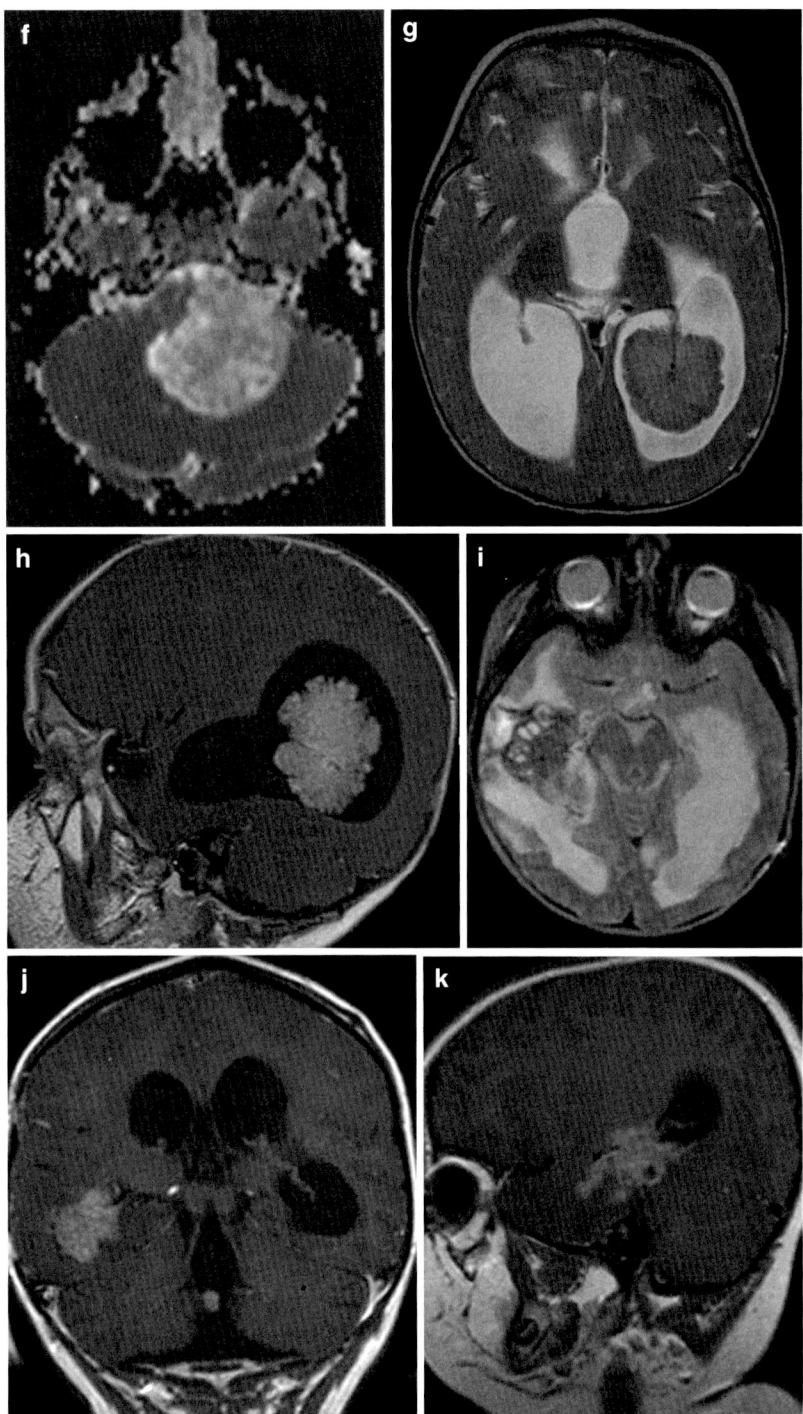

Fig. 3.26 (continued)

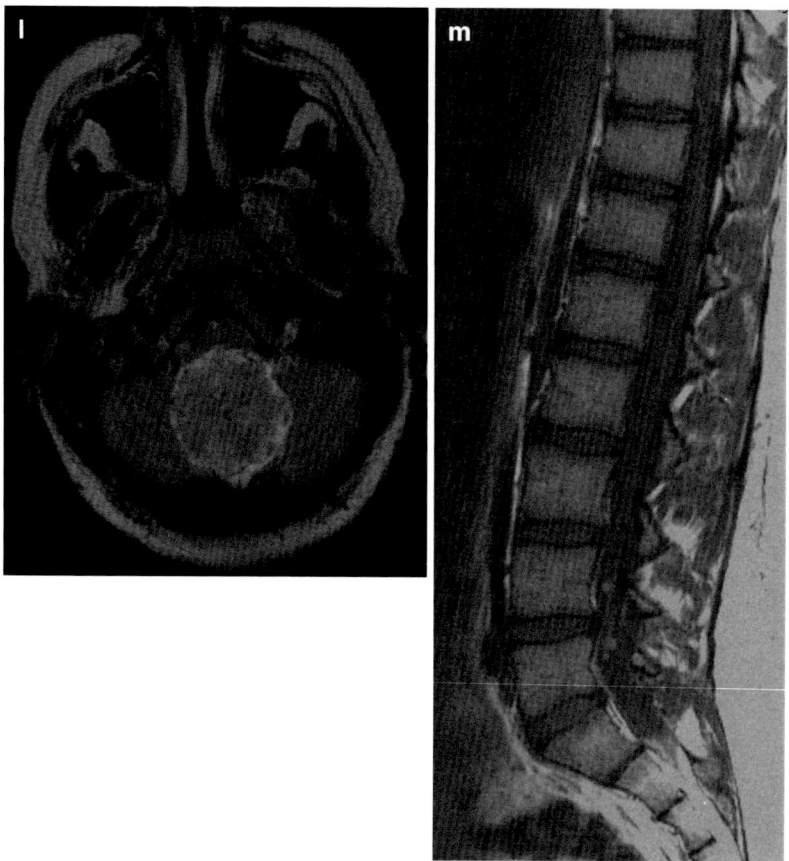

Fig. 3.26 (continued)

Chapter 4
Imaging Guidelines for Pediatric Brain Tumor Patients

4.1 Imaging Techniques

MRI is clearly the method of choice for the imaging of diseases of the CNS. CT usually has only an additional role in case of emergency or contraindications against MRI. For radiotherapy planning the physical properties of CT are essential [114]. However, it still is the only method for a reliable depiction of calcifications near the skull base, which can have a diagnostic potential in some tumor entities [115, 116]. The signal intensities on MRI and density values on CT allow a limited diagnosis of the histology of the tumor (see Chap. 3). Invasive angiography or conventional radiography is useful only in rare exceptions.

4.1.1 Standard MRI Technique (Proposal for the SIOP-E Tumor Trials)

Additional to the standard SE sequences, an increasing number of various sequences have become available. However, the imaging characteristics on these sequences and thus the size of tumors might vary artificially. Key to a correct evaluation of study patients in a comparable way is to keep standardized imaging sequences during follow-up. A standard imaging protocol should contain T2/FLAIR (or proton density PD) sequences. FLAIR alone is not sufficient, because the cell density of a tumor cannot be sufficiently evaluated without a T2-sequence. The only performance of a T2 or FLAIR bears the risk to miss pathology (Fig. 4.1a–c). They should be combined with T1-weighted sequences before and after intravenous (i.v.) administration of contrast material. For children, the slice length should not exceed 4 mm. For small structures even much smaller slice lengths might be necessary. Although many surgical or radiotherapy treatment planning systems require three-dimensional sequences, these should only be additional to the core of standard imaging, because

© Springer International Publishing Switzerland 2017 55
M. Warmuth-Metz, *Imaging and Diagnosis in Pediatric Brain Tumor Studies*,
DOI 10.1007/978-3-319-42503-0_4

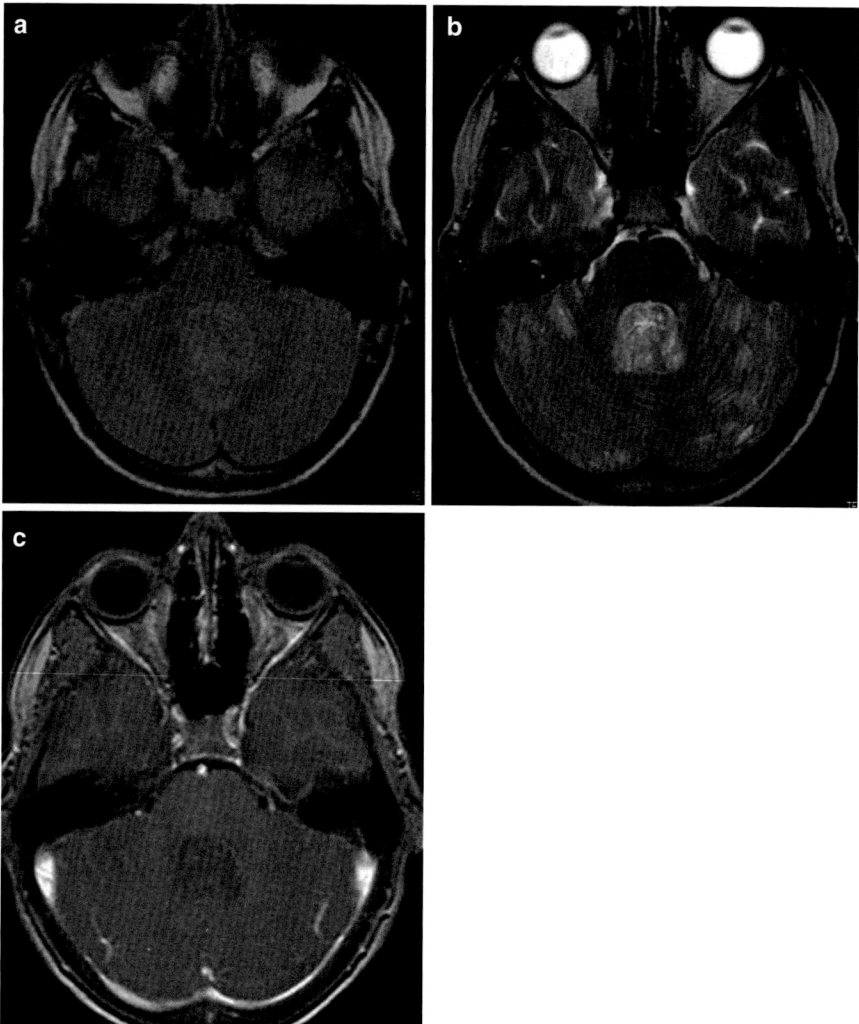

Fig. 4.1 (a–i) T2 and FLAIR of the brain are necessary for complete evaluation. While on FLAIR (**a**) there is no suspicion of dissemination, leptomeningeal deposits in the cerebellar sulci are clearly seen on T2 (**b**). On an enhanced T1 (**c**), the leptomeningeal dissemination is not detectable as well. Note the nonenhancing primary tumor (MB) in the fourth ventricle. But it may also be vice versa and it cannot be predicted in the individual case. In a child with an ependymoma the histologically verified metastases in the cerebral sulci are only visible FLAIR (**d**) but not on T2 (**e**). The comparison of a precontrast SE image (**f**) with a postcontrast MPR (**g**) for the definition of an enhancing residual tumor may be hard or even impossible. The tiny spinal metastasis is not visible on the 1 mm thick MPR sequences (**h**) while it can be clearly seen on the thicker turbo SE (TSE) series (**i**) done during the same examination

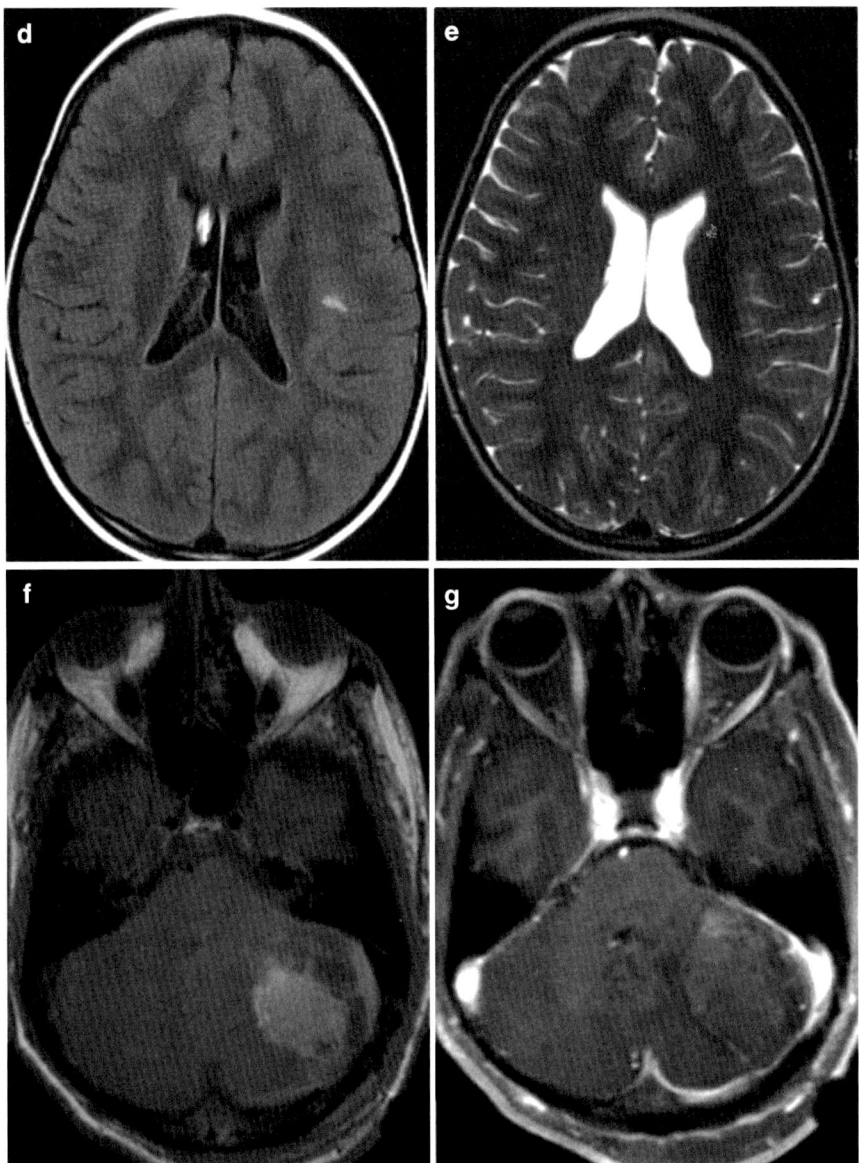

Fig. 4.1 (continued)

the contrast behavior of tumors on SE series and on 3-D-MPR series can differ considerably [117] making a comparison impossible (Fig. 4.1f–i). An automatized 3-D volume calculation of brain tumors can only be used in single or limited center studies because the acquisition parameters have to be uniform.

Diffusion weighted MRI (DWI) with the additional calculation of the ADC allows not only the depiction of infarcted brain but also an estimation of cellular density in the absence of hemorrhage [118]. Together with the signal intensity on

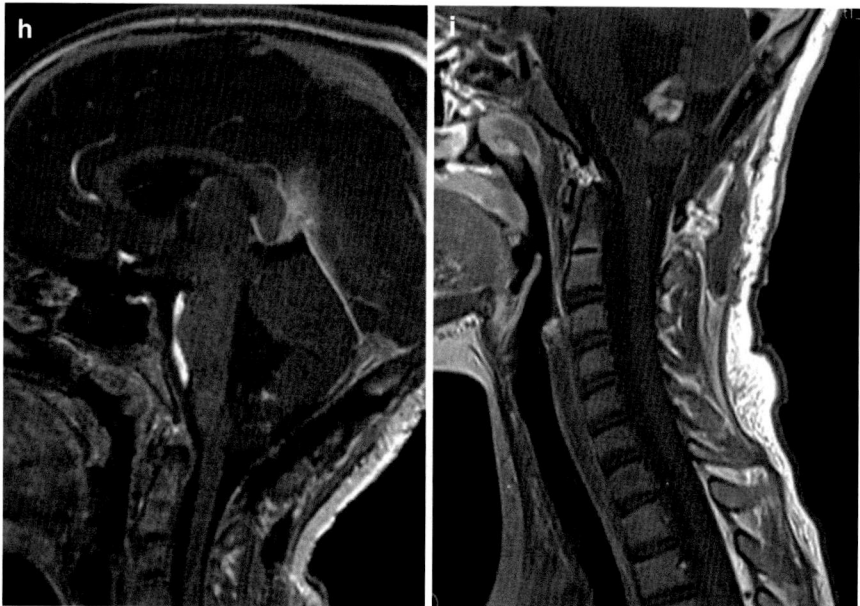

Fig. 4.1 (continued)

T2-weighted MRI the ADC is a very useful tool for differential diagnosis [119]. Susceptibility weighted sequences (SWI) are useful for the identification of calcifications or blood degradation products. However, in pediatric brain tumors with the exception of craniopharyngiomas this feature is of little importance (see also Fig. 3.9f) compared to its value in the differentiation of adult high-grade gliomas [115, 116]. As SWI sequences are prone to disturbances by susceptibility artifacts the skull base is not a useful region.

4.1.2 Early Postoperative Imaging

A residual tumor after resection can only be identified within the first 3 days after resection because after this time period a nonspecific reaction of the brain to the surgical trauma can create contrast enhancement which is virtually indistinguishable from residual tumor [120] (Fig. 4.2a–c). Unfortunately also during and very early after resection surgery induced enhancement may cause problems in the identification of a possible residual tumor especially in case of the use of electrocoagulation [121] (Fig. 4.2d–g). Therefore and because of frequent increased artifacts induced by air in the intracranial cavity (Fig. 4.2h, i), we do not advice to enter the MRI directly from the operating theatre to perform the early postoperative MRI, which seems very attractive in terms of logistics. Ideal for the early postoperative MRI are day 1 and 2 after surgery. However, if in case of a contrast enhancing tumor this time period is missed, then the correct identification of a residual tumor might not be possible for a long time or even forever (Fig. 4.2a–c). Nonenhancing tumors

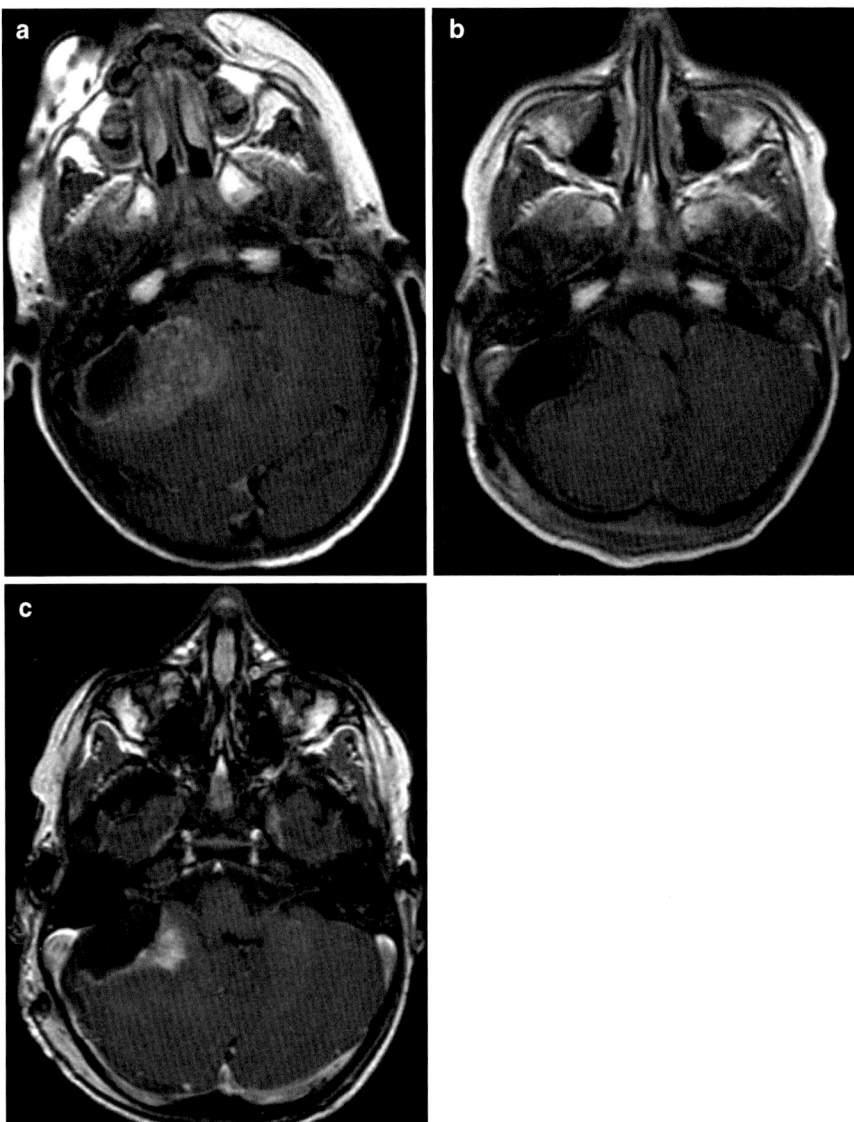

Fig. 4.2 (**a–i**) If the early postoperative time period is missed, postsurgical effects might mimic an enhancing residual tumor (**a**, morphology of a medulloblastoma on preoperative enhanced T1-weighted MRI; **b**, regular, early-postoperative MRI on day 1, enhanced T1-weighted image without residual tumor; **c**, enhanced T1-weighted MRI on day 8 after surgery with nonspecific postoperative enhancement). On very early postoperative MRI immediately after surgery, false positive enhancement possibly after coagulation during surgery may mimic a residual tumor (**d**, preoperative postcontrast T1-weighted MRI of a pilocytic astrocytoma in the vermis cerebelli; **e, f** T1-weighted pre- and postcontrast MRI immediately after surgery showing a lot of marginal enhancement also in parts of the tumor without preoperative enhancement, which is completely resolved without further treatment on the first control after 3 months (**g**)). Intracranial air can lead to heavy susceptibility artifacts on very early postoperative MRI. The sagittal T2-weighted SE image (**h**) shows a complete air filling of the ventricles and the superior parts of the subarachnoid spaces. This leads to a massive effacement on T2* images (**i**)

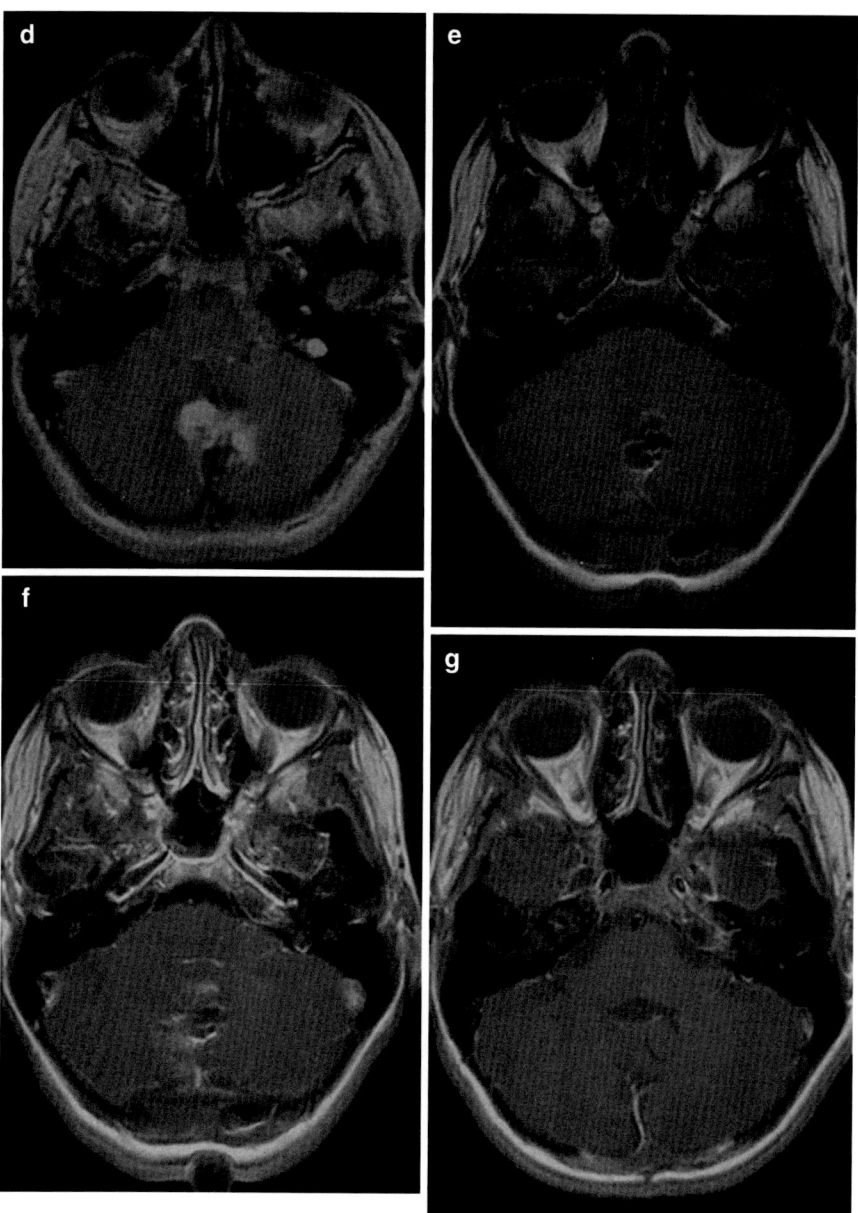

Fig. 4.2 (continued)

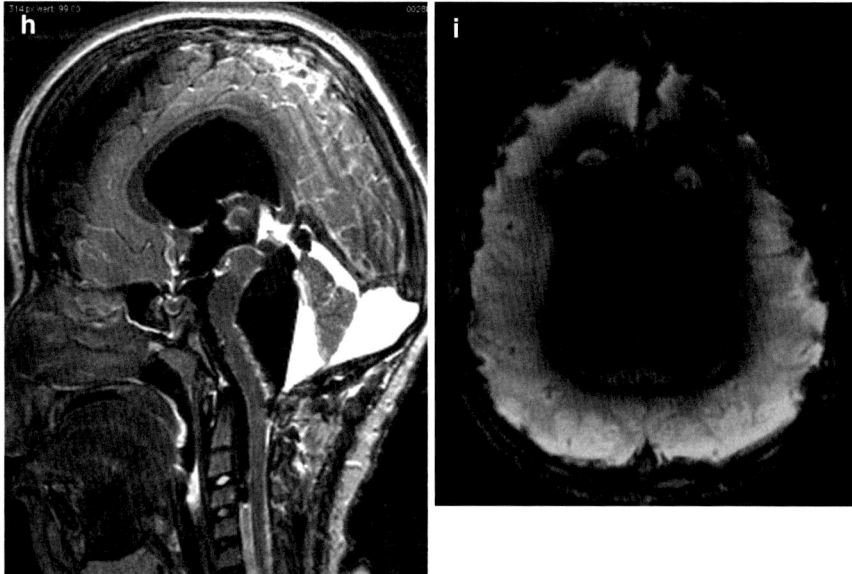

Fig. 4.2 (continued)

can only be identified on the basis of their T2/FLAIR or PD characteristics. Therefore, the comparability of MRI to the preoperative time point is of utmost importance. Also a change of magnetic field strength is problematic and should be avoided for the pre- and postoperative comparison and also for further follow-up.

4.1.3 Meningeal Dissemination

All CNS tumors can disseminate in the CSF. However, for embryonal tumors like MB, AT/RT, and ependymomas especially during follow-up, germ cell tumors, and young children with LGGs of the chiasmatic region, there is a known propensity for higher percentage of CSF seeding. In such cases, it is very useful not only to perform a cranial MRI but also to add a spinal MRI after the cranial examination has been finished. For a correct staging, the visualization of the entire dural space intracranially and in the spinal canal is necessary. MRI is the only noninvasive method for the evaluation of a leptomeningeal dissemination of tumors or a primary spinal cord tumor.

Enhancement can affect the leptomeninx and the pachymeninx. While pachymeningeal enhancement is frequently a consequence of pressure changes in the CSF space, e.g., after surgery, in case of an implanted shunting system or after lumbar punctures leptomeningeal enhancement either represents a neoplastic or inflammatory affection. Nodular enhancement of the leptomeninges is pathognomonic for nodular meningeal dissemination and only rarely can be explained by inflammation like sarcoidosis. In laminar enhancement a lumbar tab can exclude meningitis as underlying reason.

In a considerable number of children with MBs or other tumors prone to a leptomeningeal seeding, the staging examination of the spinal canal is performed after surgery. In the immediate postsurgical time period a physiological phenomenon may occur, which is called nonspecific subdural spinal enhancement. This enhancement closely resembles the MR images known from idiopathic CSF hypotension syndrome [122, 123], where the pachymeninges and not leptomeninges are affected and can easily be differentiated from the MRI characteristics of leptomeningeal dissemination [124]. Subdural enhancement must not be mixed up with leptomeningeal disease. It seems to be a dynamic process because we observed a progressive increase in T1-signal after contrast enhancement in a few patients during repetitive sequences performed during the same MR examination (Fig. 4.3a, b). Patients are always without specific symptoms. In case of extensive subdural enhancement, a leptomeningeal dissemination cannot be excluded (Fig. 4.3b) with sufficient reliability and therefore the spinal MRI has to be repeated after about 1–2 weeks. Within this time period a reduction or complete spontaneous resolution of nonspecific enhancement is to be expected. Occasionally after surgery a fluid level of nonenhancing spinal intradural blood mainly in the sacral region can be seen and resolves spontaneously as well (Fig. 4.3c–e).

For the visualization of possible spinal leptomeningeal dissemination exclusively T1 after contrast medium application is important. Rarely T2-weighted MRI is useful for the identification of small leptomeningeal nodules or in case of nonenhancing leptomeningeal dissemination. For nonenhancing dissemination, thin T2 sequences like CISS sequences seem to be promising and should be considered for the routine spinal protocol. However, as the T1-sequence after contrast is usually the last of the standard spinal MR sequences, the clinical practice in the reference evaluation of children with brain tumors has shown that these important postcontrast T1-images are very frequently deteriorated by movement artifacts in no longer compliant awake patients or by a flattening of sedation towards the expected end of the MR examination in sedated patients. We advice to focus the spinal MRI on the T1-series after contrast enhancement. The T2-weighted MRI may be added thereafter. If a fatty filum terminale is suspected, an additional T1 with fat suppression can clarify the situation. Small deposits of leptomeningeal disease may be mistaken for physiologic vessels of the spinal cord. Vessels are easily depicted if axial slices of all areas showing possible vessel enhancement on the sagittal slices are performed additionally.

Fat suppression is a useful method for the evaluation of bone tumors in the spine. However, it is not necessary for the detection and staging of spinal leptomeningeal dissemination and additionally caries the risk of artifacts rendering the images ine-

Fig. 4.3 (a–f) T1-weighted TSE series early after contrast medium application (a) shows faint subdural enhancement and a thick leptomeningeal laminar dissemination (*arrow*) on the spinal cord. This dissemination is masked on the repeat postcontrast series (b) 20 min after (a). A small fluid-fluid-level can be seen as horizontally confined structure in prone position (*arrow*) on T2 (c), T1-weighted MRI before (d) and after contrast (e). The signal is compatible with very fresh blood and this lesion vanishes within a few days. The use of fat suppression techniques for the evaluation of a spinal leptomeningeal dissemination is not necessary and not rarely impaired by artifacts mainly in the transition from the chest to the neck (f)

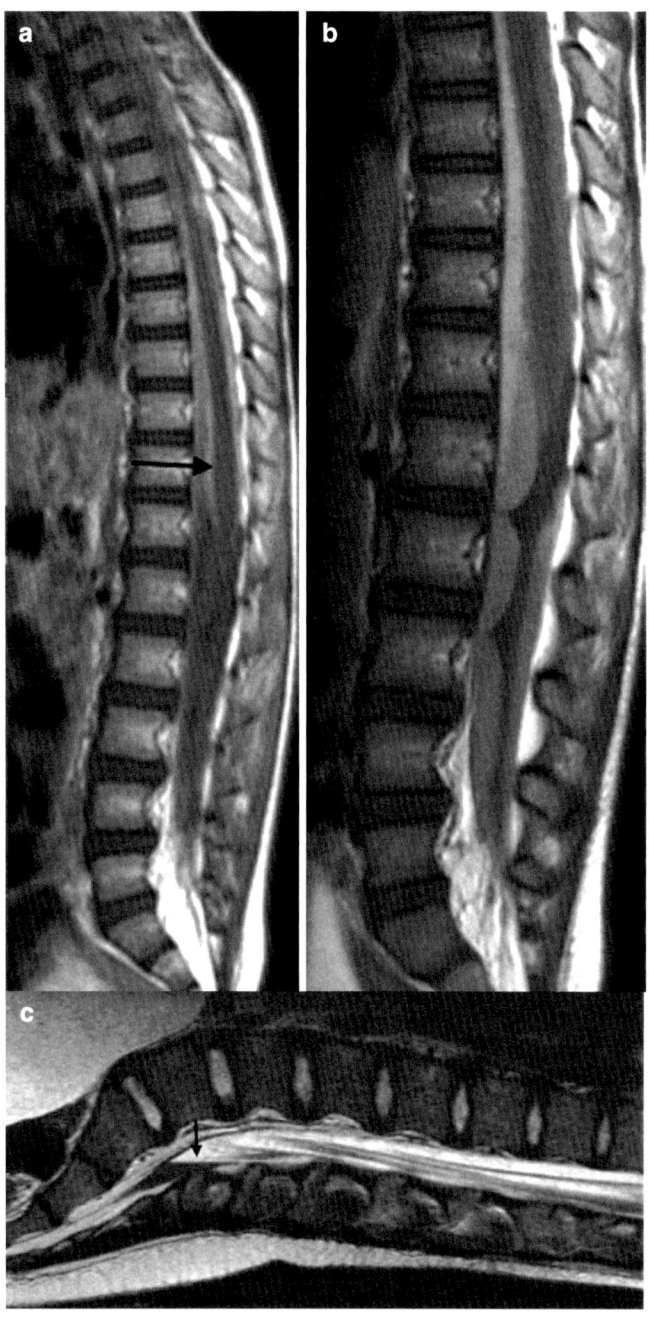

Fig. 4.3 (continued)

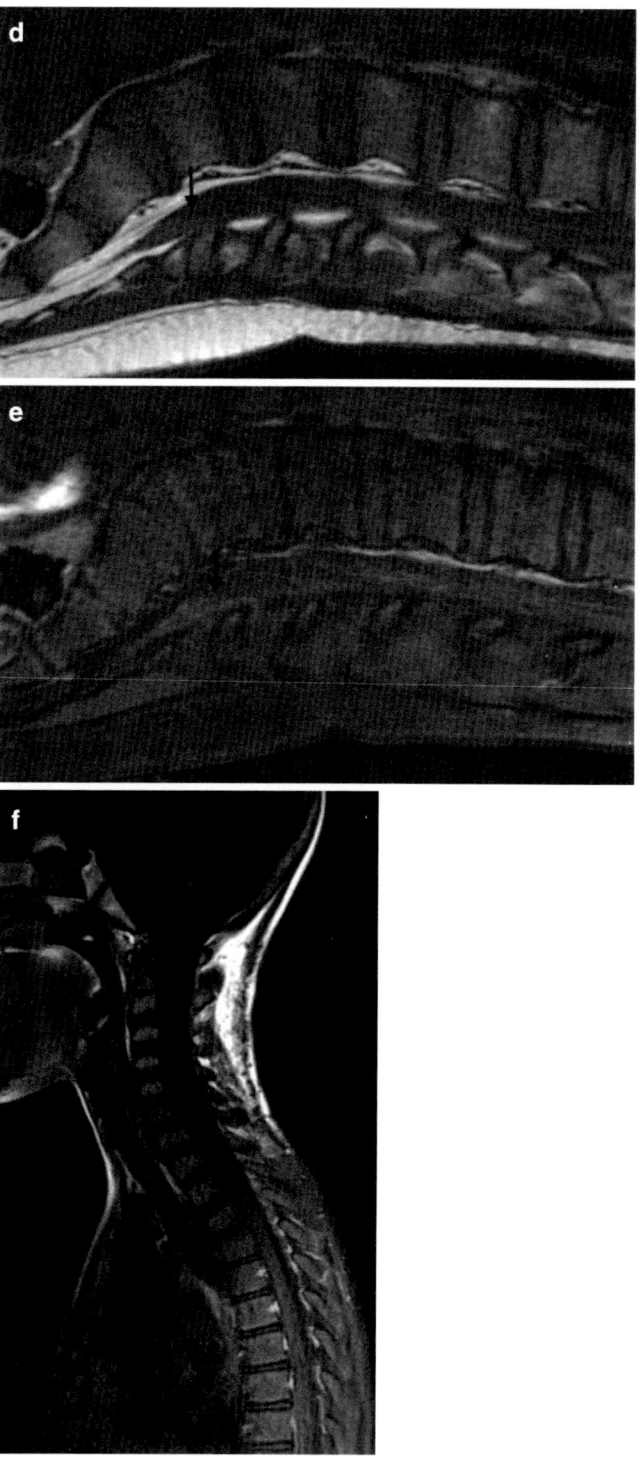

valuable mainly in the transition of the chest to the neck (Fig. 4.3f). Other artifacts like pulsations or increase of T1-signal of the CSF are more frequent in 3 T than in 1.5 T. To discriminate prominent cord veins from leptomeningeal seeding axial slices are advisable and a slice thickness of at least 4 mm is usually of better signal to noise ratio compared to extremely thin slices.

4.1.4 Follow-Up Examinations

Response of tumors is traditionally evaluated by size measurement. Therefore comparable imaging parameters have to be used to guarantee as much accuracy as possible. In tumors only measurable on T2/FLAIR images like DIPG or nonenhancing tumors, a second plane of one or both of these sequences should be provided to enable a volume calculation.

4.1.4.1 Differential Diagnosis Between Recurrence or Treatment Related Changes

In pilocytic astrocytomas, an intensification of enhancement or a new contrast enhancement must not be mistaken for a malignant degeneration and progression. In these tumors, enhancement is strongly varying and not related to prognosis with [125] and without treatment [126]. We have evaluated 83 children with measurable LGGs irrespective of treatment or during a watch-and-wait strategy according to their contrast behavior and found that in general growing tumors show increasing enhancement and vice versa. However, the groups of tumors with reduced and intensified enhancement also contained about 1/3 of tumors, which showed a contrary behavior like growing tumors with reduced enhancement and shrinking tumors with increasing enhancement. In conclusion, contrast enhancement alone is not decisive and does not mean progression in the absence of tumor growth.

New lesions like T2-hyperintensity and contrast enhancement in the brain parenchyma in embryonal tumors like MB after treatment with radiotherapy are frequently misdiagnosed as recurrence. MB and probably also the other embryonal entities and also ependymomas show two kinds of recurrences. They either recur locally in the surgical bed or as leptomeningeal dissemination or both in combination. However, we never saw a recurrence in the brain outside the surgical bed. Therefore treatment related changes like temporary (Fig. 4.4a–d) effects (early delayed reaction [127, 128]) or second tumors [129] (Fig. 4.4e, f) are much more likely than a true recurrence of the primary tumor. To raise the suspicion of a radiation reaction it has to be clarified with the radiotherapist that a sufficiently high dose has been applied to the affected region. Multimodal imaging like MR-spectroscopy, MR-perfusion, or aminoacid-PET can help in the differentiation.

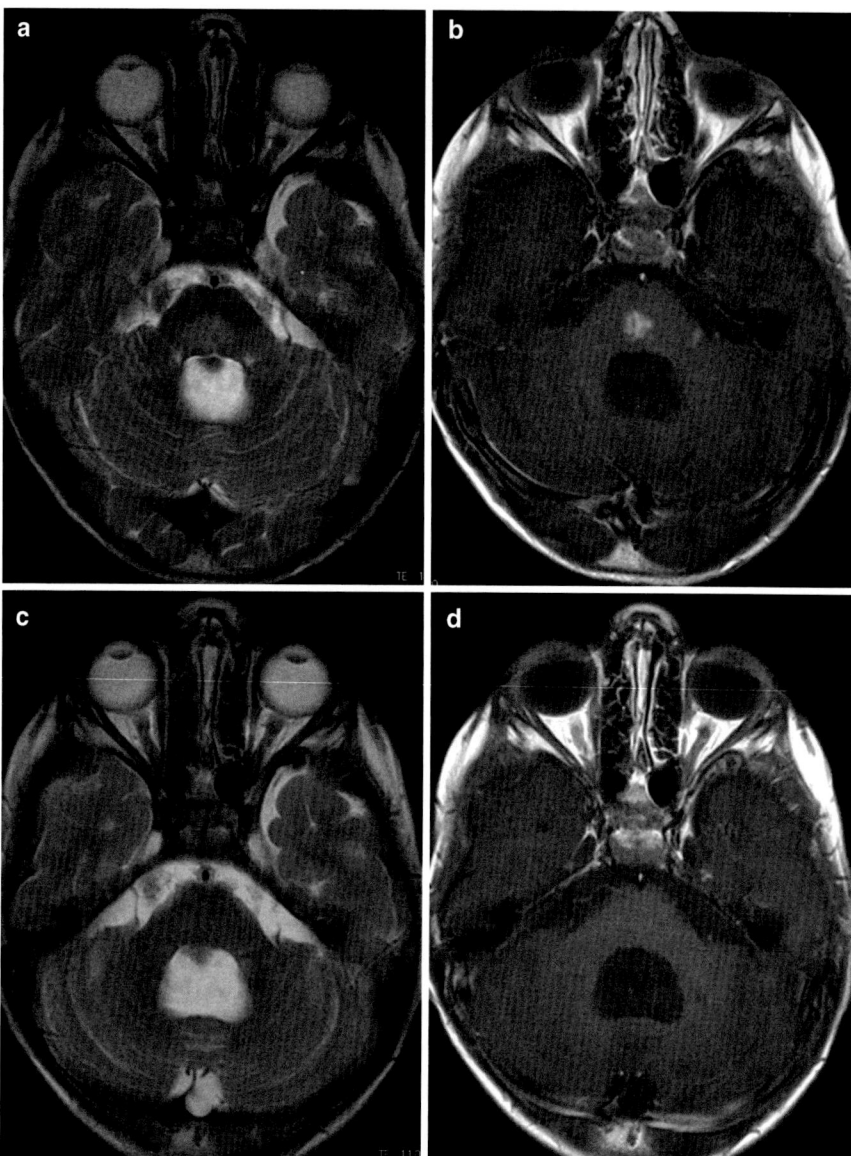

Fig. 4.4 (a–f) 9 months after complete resection of a medulloblastoma in the fourth ventricle, a new T2-lesion (**a**) with enhancement (**b**) is seen in the pons. This area was within the treatment dose area of radiation. Without specific treatment the changes vanished within 3 months of follow-up (**c, d**). However, early delayed radiation reactions may also increase or resolve more slowly. In a child, 7 years after completed treatment for a MB new and enlarging lesions developed in the cerebellum on the right hand side, the pons (**e**), and surrounding the lateral ventricles (*arrows*) with involvement of the corpus callosum and meaning subependymal spread (**f**). The histology of this second tumor was a glioblastoma

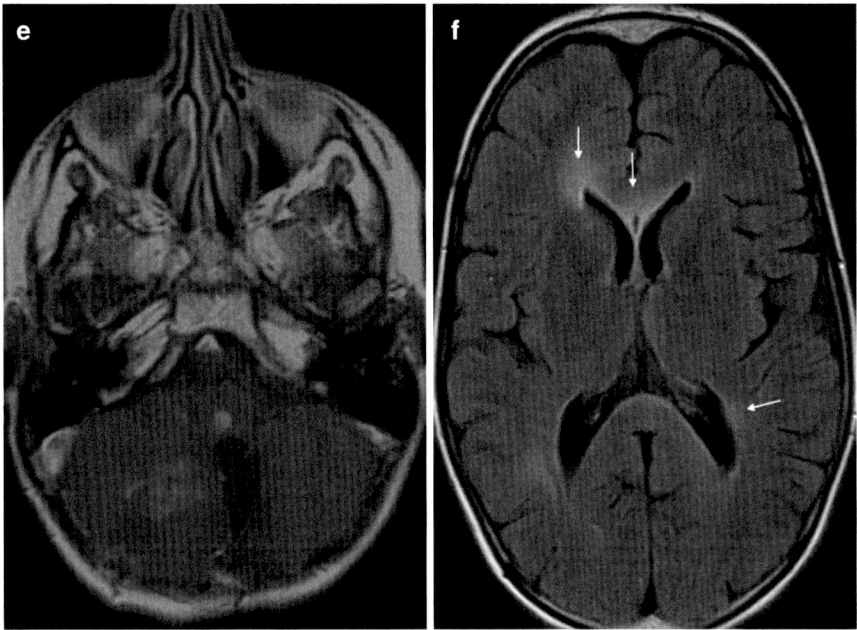

Fig. 4.4 (continued)

References

1. Northcott PA, Korshunov A, Pfister SM, Taylor MD. The clinical implications of medulloblastoma subgroups. Nat Rev Neurol. 2012;8:340–51.
2. Chang CH, Housepian EM, Herbert Jr C. An operative staging system and a megavoltage radiotherapeutic technic for cerebellar medulloblastomas. Radiology. 1969;93:1351–9.
3. Packer RJ, Gajjar A, Vezina G, et al. Phase III study of craniospinal radiation therapy followed by adjuvant chemotherapy for newly diagnosed average-risk medulloblastoma. J Clin Oncol Off J Am Soc Clin Oncol. 2006;24:4202–8.
4. Lannering B, Rutkowski S, Doz F, et al. Hyperfractionated versus conventional radiotherapy followed by chemotherapy in standard-risk medulloblastoma: results from the randomized multicenter HIT-SIOP PNET 4 trial. J Clin Oncol Off J Am Soc Clin Oncol. 2012;30: 3187–93.
5. Gajjar A, Bowers DC, Karajannis MA, Leary S, Witt H, Gottardo NG. Pediatric brain tumors: innovative genomic information is transforming the diagnostic and clinical landscape. J Clin Oncol. 2015;33:2986–98.
6. Tallen G, Resch A, Calaminus G, et al. Strategies to improve the quality of survival for childhood brain tumour survivors. Eur J Paediatr Neurol EJPN Off J Eur Paediatr Neurol Soc. 2015;19:619–39.
7. Warmuth-Metz M, Bison B, Leykamm S. Neuroradiologic review in pediatric brain tumor studies. Klin Neuroradiol. 2009;19:263–73.
8. Lannering B, Rutkowski S, Doz F, et al. Hyperfractionated versus conventional radiotherapy followed by chemotherapy in standard-risk medulloblastoma: results from the randomized multicenter HIT-SIOP PNET 4 trial. J Clin Oncol. 2012;30:3187–93.
9. Louis DN, Perry A, Reifenberger G, et al. The 2016 World Health Organization Classification of Tumors of the Central Nervous System: a summary. Acta Neuropathol 2016;131: 803–820.
10. Rorke LB, Trojanowski JQ, Lee VM, et al. Primitive neuroectodermal tumors of the central nervous system. Brain Pathol. 1997;7:765–84.
11. Louis DN, Ohgaki H, Wiestler OD, et al. The 2007 WHO classification of tumours of the central nervous system. Acta Neuropathol. 2007;114:97–109.
12. Ramaswamy V, Remke M, Bouffet E, et al. Risk stratification of childhood medulloblastoma in the molecular era: the current consensus. Acta Neuropathol. 2016;131:821–31.
13. Anderson AW, Xie J, Pizzonia J, Bronen RA, Spencer DD, Gore JC. Effects of cell volume fraction changes on apparent diffusion in human cells. Magn Reson Imaging. 2000;18:689–95.
14. Tortori-Donati P, Fondelli MP, Rossi A, et al. Medulloblastoma in children: CT and MRI findings. Neuroradiology. 1996;38:352–9.

© Springer International Publishing Switzerland 2017
M. Warmuth-Metz, *Imaging and Diagnosis in Pediatric Brain Tumor Studies*,
DOI 10.1007/978-3-319-42503-0

15. Giangaspero F, Perilongo G, Fondelli MP, et al. Medulloblastoma with extensive nodularity: a variant with favorable prognosis. J Neurosurg. 1999;91:971–7.
16. Northcott PA, Hielscher T, Dubuc A, et al. Pediatric and adult sonic hedgehog medulloblastomas are clinically and molecularly distinct. Acta Neuropathol. 2011;122:231–40.
17. Giangaspero FE, Haapasalo H, Pietsch T, Westler OD, Ellison DW. WHO classification of tumors of the central nervous system. Lyon: International Agency for Resaerch on Cancer; 2007.
18. von Hoff K, Hartmann W, von Bueren AO, et al. Large cell/anaplastic medulloblastoma: outcome according to myc status, histopathological, and clinical risk factors. Pediatr Blood Cancer. 2010;54:369–76.
19. Buhren J, Christoph AH, Buslei R, Albrecht S, Wiestler OD, Pietsch T. Expression of the neurotrophin receptor p75NTR in medulloblastomas is correlated with distinct histological and clinical features: evidence for a medulloblastoma subtype derived from the external granule cell layer. J Neuropathol Exp Neurol. 2000;59:229–40.
20. Koeller KK, Rushing EJ. From the archives of the AFIP: medulloblastoma: a comprehensive review with radiologic-pathologic correlation. Radiographics. 2003;23:1613–37.
21. Fruehwald-Pallamar J, Puchner SB, Rossi A, et al. Magnetic resonance imaging spectrum of medulloblastoma. Neuroradiology. 2011;53:387–96.
22. Garre ML, Cama A, Bagnasco F, et al. Medulloblastoma variants: age-dependent occurrence and relation to Gorlin syndrome – a new clinical perspective. Clin Cancer Res. 2009;15:2463–71.
23. Perreault S, Ramaswamy V, Achrol AS, et al. MRI surrogates for molecular subgroups of medulloblastoma. AJNR Am J Neuroradiol. 2014;35:1263–9.
24. Maher ER, Yates JR, Ferguson-Smith MA. Statistical analysis of the two stage mutation model in von Hippel-Lindau disease, and in sporadic cerebellar haemangioblastoma and renal cell carcinoma. J Med Genet. 1990;27:311–4.
25. Schittenhelm J, Nagel C, Meyermann R, Beschorner R. Atypical teratoid/rhabdoid tumors may show morphological and immunohistochemical features seen in choroid plexus tumors. Neuropathology. 2011;31:461–7.
26. Benesch M, Sperl D, von Bueren AO, et al. Primary central nervous system primitive neuroectodermal tumors (CNS-PNETs) of the spinal cord in children: four cases from the German HIT database with a critical review of the literature. J Neurooncol. 2011;104:279–86.
27. Nowak J, Seidel C, Pietsch T, et al. Systematic comparison of MRI findings in pediatric ependymoblastoma with ependymoma and CNS primitive neuroectodermal tumor not otherwise specified. Neuro Oncol. 2015;17:1157–65.
28. Woehrer A, Slavc I, Waldhoer T, et al. Incidence of atypical teratoid/rhabdoid tumors in children: a population-based study by the Austrian Brain Tumor Registry, 1996–2006. Cancer. 2010;116:5725–32.
29. von Hoff K, Hinkes B, Dannenmann-Stern E, et al. Frequency, risk-factors and survival of children with atypical teratoid rhabdoid tumors (AT/RT) of the CNS diagnosed between 1988 and 2004, and registered to the German HIT database. Pediatr Blood Cancer. 2011;57:978–85.
30. Fruhwald MC, Rickert CH, O'Dorisio MS, et al. Somatostatin receptor subtype 2 is expressed by supratentorial primitive neuroectodermal tumors of childhood and can be targeted for somatostatin receptor imaging. Clin Cancer Res Off J Am Assoc Cancer Res. 2004;10:2997–3006.
31. Bruggers CS, Bleyl SB, Pysher T, et al. Clinicopathologic comparison of familial versus sporadic atypical teratoid/rhabdoid tumors (AT/RT) of the central nervous system. Pediatr Blood Cancer. 2011;56:1026–31.
32. Warmuth-Metz M, Bison B, Dannemann-Stern E, Kortmann R, Rutkowski S, Pietsch T. CT and MR imaging in atypical teratoid/rhabdoid tumors of the central nervous system. Neuroradiology. 2008;50:447–52.
33. Dufour C, Beaugrand A, Le Deley MC, et al. Clinicopathologic prognostic factors in childhood atypical teratoid and rhabdoid tumor of the central nervous system: a multicenter study. Cancer. 2012;118:3812–21.

34. Stabouli S, Sdougka M, Tsitspoulos P, et al. Primary atypical teratoid/rhabdoid tumor of the spine in an infant. Hippokratia. 2010;14:286–8.
35. Arslanoglu A, Aygun N, Tekhtani D, et al. Imaging findings of CNS atypical teratoid/rhabdoid tumors. AJNR Am J Neuroradiol. 2004;25:476–80.
36. Warmuth-Metz M, Bison B, Gerber NU, Pietsch T, Hasselblatt M, Fruhwald MC. Bone involvement in atypical teratoid/rhabdoid tumors of the CNS. AJNR Am J Neuroradiol. 2013;34:2039–42.
37. Stagno V, Mugamba J, Ssenyonga P, Kaaya BN, Warf BC. Presentation, pathology, and treatment outcome of brain tumors in 172 consecutive children at CURE Children's Hospital of Uganda. The predominance of the visible diagnosis and the uncertainties of epidemiology in sub-Saharan Africa. Child's Nerv Syst ChNS Off J Int Soc Pediatr Neurosurg. 2014;30:137–46.
38. Fernandez C, Figarella-Branger D, Girard N, et al. Pilocytic astrocytomas in children: prognostic factors – a retrospective study of 80 cases. Neurosurgery. 2003;53:544–53; discussion 554–545.
39. Houten JK, Cooper PR. Spinal cord astrocytomas: presentation, management and outcome. J Neurooncol. 2000;47:219–24.
40. Kumar AJ, Leeds NE, Kumar VA, et al. Magnetic resonance imaging features of pilocytic astrocytoma of the brain mimicking high-grade gliomas. J Comput Assist Tomogr. 2010;34:601–11.
41. Zeng L, Liang P, Jiao J, Chen J, Lei T. Will an asymptomatic meningioma grow or Not grow? A meta-analysis. J Neurol Surg Part A Central Eur Neurosurg. 2015;76:341–7.
42. Pikis S, Cohen JE, Vargas AA, Gomori JM, Harnof S, Itshayek E. Superficial siderosis of the central nervous system secondary to spinal ependymoma. J Clin Neurosci. 2014;21:2017–9.
43. Fanous AA, Jost GF, Schmidt MH. A nonenhancing world health organization grade II intramedullary spinal ependymoma in the Conus: case illustration and review of imaging characteristics. Glob Spine J. 2012;2:57–64.
44. Cosnard G, Duprez T, Grandin C, Hernalsteen D. Intramedullary tumours and pseudotumours. J Radiol. 2010;91:988–97.
45. Listernick R, Ferner RE, Liu GT, Gutmann DH. Optic pathway gliomas in neurofibromatosis-1: controversies and recommendations. Ann Neurol. 2007;61:189–98.
46. Legius E, Descheemaeker MJ, Fryns JP, Van den Berghe H. Neurofibromatosis type 1. Genet Couns. 1994;5:225–41.
47. Dodge Jr HW, Love JG, Craig WM, et al. Gliomas of the optic nerves. AMA Arch Neurol Psychiatry. 1958;79:607–21.
48. Grill J, Laithier V, Rodriguez D, Raquin MA, Pierre-Kahn A, Kalifa C. When do children with optic pathway tumours need treatment? An oncological perspective in 106 patients treated in a single centre. Eur J Pediatr. 2000;159:692–6.
49. Taylor T, Jaspan T, Milano G, et al. Radiological classification of optic pathway gliomas: experience of a modified functional classification system. Br J Radiol. 2008;81:761–6.
50. Kearney D, Tay-Kearney ML, Khangure MS. Craniopharyngioma and the moustache sign. Australas Radiol. 1993;37:370–1.
51. Saeki N, Uchino Y, Murai H, et al. MR imaging study of edema-like change along the optic tract in patients with pituitary region tumors. AJNR Am J Neuroradiol. 2003;24:336–42.
52. Wong JY, Uhl V, Wara WM, Sheline GE. Optic gliomas. A reanalysis of the University of California, San Francisco experience. Cancer. 1987;60:1847–55.
53. Frohman LP, Guirgis M, Turbin RE, Bielory L. Sarcoidosis of the anterior visual pathway: 24 new cases. J Neuroophthalmol Off J N Am Neuroophthalmol Soc. 2003;23:190–7.
54. Ng KL, McDermott N, Romanowski CA, Jackson A. Neurosarcoidosis masquerading as glioma of the optic chiasm in a child. Postgrad Med J. 1995;71:265–8.
55. Cote M, Salzman KL, Sorour M, Couldwell WT. Normal dimensions of the posterior pituitary bright spot on magnetic resonance imaging. J Neurosurg. 2014;120:357–62.
56. Tao Y, Lian D, Hui-juan Z, Hui P, Zi-meng J. Value of brain magnetic resonance imaging and tumor markers in the diagnosis and treatment of intracranial germinoma in children. Zhongguo Yi Xue Ke Xue Yuan Xue Bao Acta Acad Med Sin. 2011;33:111–5.

57. Kilday JP, Laughlin S, Urbach S, Bouffet E, Bartels U. Diabetes insipidus in pediatric germinomas of the suprasellar region: characteristic features and significance of the pituitary bright spot. J Neurooncol. 2015;121:167–75.

58. Nam DH, Wang KC, Shin CH, Yang SW, Cho BK. A simple method of predicting hormonal outcome in children with intracranial germinoma. Child's Nerv Syst ChNS Off J Int Soc Pediatr Neurosurg. 1999;15:179–84.

59. Crotty TB, Scheithauer BW, Young Jr WF, et al. Papillary craniopharyngioma: a clinicopathological study of 48 cases. J Neurosurg. 1995;83:206–14.

60. Fujimaki T, Matsutani M, Funada N, et al. CT and MRI features of intracranial germ cell tumors. J Neurooncol. 1994;19:217–26.

61. Liang L, Korogi Y, Sugahara T, et al. MRI of intracranial germ-cell tumours. Neuroradiology. 2002;44:382–8.

62. Fuller GN, Kros JM. Gliomatosis cerebri. In: Louis DN, Ohgaki H, Wiestler O, Cavanee WK, editors. WHO classification of tumors of the central nervous system. Lyon: IARC; 2007.

63. Yang S, Wetzel S, Law M, Zagzag D, Cha S. Dynamic contrast-enhanced T2*-weighted MR imaging of gliomatosis cerebri. AJNR Am J Neuroradiol. 2002;23:350–5.

64. Duncan GG, Goodman GB, Ludgate CM, Rheaume DE. The treatment of adult supratentorial high grade astrocytomas. J Neurooncol. 1992;13:63–72.

65. Ampil F, Burton GV, Gonzalez-Toledo E, Nanda A. Do we need whole brain irradiation in multifocal or multicentric high-grade cerebral gliomas? Review of cases and the literature. J Neurooncol. 2007;85:353–5.

66. Broadway SJ, Ogg RJ, Scoggins MA, Sanford R, Patay Z, Boop FA. Surgical management of tumors producing the thalamopeduncular syndrome of childhood. J Neurosurg Pediatr. 2011;7:589–95.

67. Tomita T, Cortes RF. Astrocytomas of the cerebral peduncle in children: surgical experience in seven patients. Childs Nerv Syst. 2002;18:225–30.

68. Griessenauer CJ, Rizk E, Miller JH, et al. Pediatric tectal plate gliomas: clinical and radiological progression, MR imaging characteristics, and management of hydrocephalus. J Neurosurg Pediatr. 2014;13:13–20.

69. Poussaint TY, Kowal JR, Barnes PD, et al. Tectal tumors of childhood: clinical and imaging follow-up. AJNR Am J Neuroradiol. 1998;19:977–83.

70. Puget S, Philippe C, Bax DA, et al. Mesenchymal transition and PDGFRA amplification/mutation are key distinct oncogenic events in pediatric diffuse intrinsic pontine gliomas. PLoS One. 2012;7, e30313.

71. Castel D, Philippe C, Calmon R, et al. Histone H3F3A and HIST1H3B K27M mutations define two subgroups of diffuse intrinsic pontine gliomas with different prognosis and phenotypes. Acta Neuropathol. 2015;130:815–27.

72. Fischbein NJ, Prados MD, Wara W, Russo C, Edwards MS, Barkovich AJ. Radiologic classification of brain stem tumors: correlation of magnetic resonance imaging appearance with clinical outcome. Pediatr Neurosurg. 1996;24:9–23.

73. Jansen MH, Veldhuijzen van Zanten SE, Sanchez Aliaga E, et al. Survival prediction model of children with diffuse intrinsic pontine glioma based on clinical and radiological criteria. Neuro Oncol. 2015;17:160–6.

74. Hipp SJ, Steffen-Smith E, Hammoud D, Shih JH, Bent R, Warren KE. Predicting outcome of children with diffuse intrinsic pontine gliomas using multiparametric imaging. Neuro Oncol. 2011;13:904–9.

75. Sethi R, Allen J, Donahue B, et al. Prospective neuraxis MRI surveillance reveals a high risk of leptomeningeal dissemination in diffuse intrinsic pontine glioma. J Neurooncol. 2011;102:121–7.

76. Hoffman LM, DeWire M, Ryall S, et al. Spatial genomic heterogeneity in diffuse intrinsic pontine and midline high-grade glioma: implications for diagnostic biopsy and targeted therapeutics. Acta Neuropathol Commun. 2016;4:1.

77. Ghodsi M, Mortazavi A, Shahjouei S, et al. Exophytic glioma of the medulla: presentation, management and outcome. Pediatr Neurosurg. 2013;49:195–201.

78. Fisher PG, Breiter SN, Carson BS, et al. A clinicopathologic reappraisal of brain stem tumor classification. Identification of pilocystic astrocytoma and fibrillary astrocytoma as distinct entities. Cancer. 2000;89:1569–76.

79. Schneider D, Monoranu CM, Huang B, et al. Pediatric supratentorial ependymomas show more frequent deletions on chromosome 9 than infratentorial ependymomas: a microsatellite analysis. Cancer Genet Cytogenet. 2009;191:90–6.

80. Yuh EL, Barkovich AJ, Gupta N. Imaging of ependymomas: MRI and CT. Childs Nerv Syst. 2009;25:1203–13.

81. Osborn AG. Non-astrocytic neoplasms. In: Osborn's Brain. Imaging, Pathology, and Anatomy. 1st ed. Amirsys; 493–521.

82. Armington WG, Osborn AG, Cubberley DA, et al. Supratentorial ependymoma: CT appearance. Radiology. 1985;157:367–72.

83. Furie DM, Provenzale JM. Supratentorial ependymomas and subependymomas: CT and MR appearance. J Comput Assist Tomogr. 1995;19:518–26.

84. Rezai AR, Woo HH, Lee M, Cohen H, Zagzag D, Epstein FJ. Disseminated ependymomas of the central nervous system. J Neurosurg. 1996;85:618–24.

85. Bandopadhayay P, Silvera VM, Ciarlini PD, et al. Myxopapillary ependymomas in children: imaging, treatment and outcomes. J Neurooncol. 2016;126:165–74.

86. Shirasawa H, Ishii K, Iwanami A, et al. Pediatric myxopapillary ependymoma treated with subtotal resection and radiation therapy: a case report and review of the literature. Spinal Cord. 2014;52 Suppl 2:S18–20.

87. Lee D, Suh YL. Histologically confirmed intracranial germ cell tumors; an analysis of 62 patients in a single institute. Virchows Archiv Int J Pathol. 2010;457:347–57.

88. Ogiwara H, Tsutsumi Y, Matsuoka K, Kiyotani C, Terashima K, Morota N. Apparent diffusion coefficient of intracranial germ cell tumors. J Neurooncol. 2015;121:565–71.

89. Ozelame RV, Shroff M, Wood B, et al. Basal ganglia germinoma in children with associated ipsilateral cerebral and brain stem hemiatrophy. Pediatr Radiol. 2006;36:325–30.

90. Cuccia V, Alderete D. Suprasellar/pineal bifocal germ cell tumors. Childs Nerv Syst. 2010;26:1043–9.

91. Takahashi S, Yoshida K, Kawase T. Intracranial germ cell tumors: efficacy of neoadjuvant chemo-radiotherapy without surgical biopsy. Keio J Med. 2011;60:56–64.

92. Calaminus G, Bamberg M, Jurgens H, et al. Impact of surgery, chemotherapy and irradiation on long term outcome of intracranial malignant non-germinomatous germ cell tumors: results of the German Cooperative Trial MAKEI 89. Klin Padiatr. 2004;216:141–9.

93. Reisch N, Kuhne-Eversmann L, Franke D, et al. Intracranial germinoma as a very rare cause of panhypopituitarism in a 23-year old man. Exp Clin Endocrinol Diabetes. 2009;117:320–3.

94. Janmohamed S, Grossman AB, Metcalfe K, et al. Suprasellar germ cell tumours: specific problems and the evolution of optimal management with a combined chemoradiotherapy regimen. Clin Endocrinol (Oxf). 2002;57:487–500.

95. Jennings MT, Gelman R, Hochberg F. Intracranial germ-cell tumors: natural history and pathogenesis. J Neurosurg. 1985;63:155–67.

96. Jorsal T, Rorth M. Intracranial germ cell tumours. A review with special reference to endocrine manifestations. Acta Oncol. 2012;51:3–9.

97. Kreutz J, Rausin L, Weerts E, Tebache M, Born J, Hoyoux C. Intracranial germ cell tumor. JBR-BTR. 2010;93:196–7.

98. Ghirardello S, Garre ML, Rossi A, Maghnie M. The diagnosis of children with central diabetes insipidus. J Pediatr Endocrinol Metab. 2007;20:359–75.

99. Bunin GR, Surawicz TS, Witman PA, Preston-Martin S, Davis F, Bruner JM. The descriptive epidemiology of craniopharyngioma. J Neurosurg. 1998;89:547–51.

100. di Iorgi N, Secco A, Napoli F, Calandra E, Rossi A, Maghnie M. Developmental abnormalities of the posterior pituitary gland. Endocr Dev. 2009;14:83–94.

101. Schmalisch K, Beschorner R, Psaras T, Honegger J. Postoperative intracranial seeding of craniopharyngiomas – report of three cases and review of the literature. Acta Neurochir (Wien). 2010;152:313–9; discussion 319.

102. Johnson LN, Hepler RS, Yee RD, Frazee JG, Simons KB. Magnetic resonance imaging of craniopharyngioma. Am J Ophthalmol. 1986;102:242–4.

103. Muller HL, Emser A, Faldum A, et al. Longitudinal study on growth and body mass index before and after diagnosis of childhood craniopharyngioma. J Clin Endocrinol Metab. 2004;89:3298–305.

104. Paulus W, Honegger J, Keyvani K, Fahlbusch R. Xanthogranuloma of the sellar region: a clinicopathological entity different from adamantinomatous craniopharyngioma. Acta Neuropathol. 1999;97:377–82.

105. Kamoshima Y, Sawamura Y, Motegi H, Kubota K, Houkin K. Xanthogranuloma of the sellar region of children: series of five cases and literature review. Neurol Med Chir (Tokyo). 2011;51:689–93.

106. Elliott RE, Moshel YA, Wisoff JH. Minimal residual calcification and recurrence after gross-total resection of craniopharyngioma in children. J Neurosurg Pediatr. 2009;3:276–83.

107. Muller HL, Gebhardt U, Teske C, et al. Post-operative hypothalamic lesions and obesity in childhood craniopharyngioma: results of the multinational prospective trial KRANIOPHARYNGEOM 2000 after 3-year follow-up. Eur J Endocrinol. 2011;165:17–24.

108. Muller HL. Risk-adapted treatment and follow-up management in childhood-onset craniopharyngioma. Expert Rev Neurother. 2016;16:535–48.

109. Puget S, Garnett M, Wray A, et al. Pediatric craniopharyngiomas: classification and treatment according to the degree of hypothalamic involvement. J Neurosurg. 2007;106:3–12.

110. de Vile CJ, Grant DB, Hayward RD, Kendall BE, Neville BG, Stanhope R. Obesity in childhood craniopharyngioma: relation to post-operative hypothalamic damage shown by magnetic resonance imaging. J Clin Endocrinol Metab. 1996;81:2734–7.

111. Janisch W, Staneczek W. Primary tumors of the choroid plexus. Frequency, localization and age. Zentralbl Allg Pathol Pathologische Anatomie. 1989;135:235–40.

112. Guermazi A, De Kerviler E, Zagdanski AM, Frija J. Diagnostic imaging of choroid plexus disease. Clin Radiol. 2000;55:503–16.

113. Meyers SP, Khademian ZP, Chuang SH, Pollack IF, Korones DN, Zimmerman RA. Choroid plexus carcinomas in children: MRI features and patient outcomes. Neuroradiology. 2004;46:770–80.

114. Stephenson JA, Wiley Jr AL. Current techniques in three-dimensional CT simulation and radiation treatment planning. Oncology. 1995;9:1225–32, 1235; discussion 1235–1240.

115. Zulfiqar M, Dumrongpisutikul N, Intrapiromkul J, Yousem DM. Detection of intratumoral calcification in oligodendrogliomas by susceptibility-weighted MR imaging. AJNR Am J Neuroradiol. 2012;33:858–64.

116. Tsuda M, Takahashi S, Higano S, Kurihara N, Ikeda H, Sakamoto K. CT and MR imaging of craniopharyngioma. Eur Radiol. 1997;7:464–9.

117. Kato Y, Higano S, Tamura H, et al. Usefulness of contrast-enhanced T1-weighted sampling perfection with application-optimized contrasts by using different flip angle evolutions in detection of small brain metastasis at 3 T MR imaging: comparison with magnetization-prepared rapid acquisition of gradient echo imaging. AJNR Am J Neuroradiol. 2009;30:923–9.

118. Kan P, Liu JK, Hedlund G, Brockmeyer DL, Walker ML, Kestle JR. The role of diffusion-weighted magnetic resonance imaging in pediatric brain tumors. Child's Nerv Syst ChNS Off J Int Soc Pediatr Neurosurg. 2006;22:1435–9.

119. Poretti A, Meoded A, Huisman TA. Neuroimaging of pediatric posterior fossa tumors including review of the literature. J Magn Reson Imaging. 2012;35:32–47.

120. Forsting M, Albert FK, Kunze S, Adams HP, Zenner D, Sartor K. Extirpation of glioblastomas: MR and CT follow-up of residual tumor and regrowth patterns. AJNR Am J Neuroradiol. 1993;14:77–87.

121. Knauth M, Aras N, Wirtz CR, Dorfler A, Engelhorn T, Sartor K. Surgically induced intracranial contrast enhancement: potential source of diagnostic error in intraoperative MR imaging. AJNR Am J Neuroradiol. 1999;20:1547–53.
122. Kumar N, Miller GM, Piepgras DG, Mokri B. A unifying hypothesis for a patient with superficial siderosis, low-pressure headache, intraspinal cyst, back pain, and prominent vascularity. J Neurosurg. 2010;113:97–101.
123. Medina JH, Abrams K, Falcone S, Bhatia RG. Spinal imaging findings in spontaneous intracranial hypotension. AJR Am J Roentgenol. 2010;195:459–64.
124. Warmuth-Metz M, Kuhl J, Krauss J, Solymosi L. Subdural enhancement on postoperative spinal MRI after resection of posterior cranial fossa tumours. Neuroradiology. 2004;46:219–23.
125. Lesniak MS, Klem JM, Weingart J, Carson Sr BS. Surgical outcome following resection of contrast-enhanced pediatric brainstem gliomas. Pediatr Neurosurg. 2003;39:314–22.
126. Gaudino S, Quaglio F, Schiarelli C, et al. Spontaneous modifications of contrast enhancement in childhood non-cerebellar pilocytic astrocytomas. Neuroradiology. 2012;54:989–95.
127. Fouladi M, Chintagumpala M, Laningham FH, et al. White matter lesions detected by magnetic resonance imaging after radiotherapy and high-dose chemotherapy in children with medulloblastoma or primitive neuroectodermal tumor. J Clin Oncol. 2004;22:4551–60.
128. Jellinger K. Human central nervous system lesions following radiation therapy. Zentralbl Neurochir. 1977;38:199–200.
129. You SH, Lyu CJ, Kim DS, Suh CO. Second primary brain tumors following cranial irradiation for pediatric solid brain tumors. Childs Nerv Syst. 2013;29:1865–70.

Index

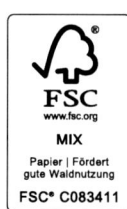